Grandma
Gail,

The Animal/Human
Bond heals where
medicine Qualters.

God Bless You   Mary Tracy
5/18/2019

Bunny Boy and Me

My Triumph over Chronic Pain with the Help of
the World's Unluckiest, Luckiest Rabbit

Nancy Laracy
Foreword by Dr. Cheryl Welch, VMD

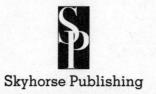

Skyhorse Publishing

Skyhorse Publishing books may be purchased in bulk at special discounts for sales promotion, corporate gifts, fund-raising, or educational purposes. Special editions can also be created to specifications. For details, contact the Special Sales Department, Skyhorse Publishing, 307 West 36th Street, 11th Floor, New York, NY 10018 or info@skyhorsepublishing.com.

Skyhorse® and Skyhorse Publishing® are registered trademarks of Skyhorse Publishing, Inc.®, a Delaware corporation.

Visit our website at www.skyhorsepublishing.com.

10 9 8 7 6 5 4 3 2 1

Library of Congress Cataloging-in-Publication Data is available on file.

Cover design by Mona Lin
Cover photo credit Nancy Laracy

Print ISBN: 978-1-5107-3682-5
Ebook ISBN: 978-1-5107-3683-2

Printed in the United States of America

This book is dedicated to **Cheryl Welch, VMD,** and **Bunny Boy** who have no doubt been reunited on the other side of the Rainbow Bridge. They both left huge footprints to fill during their time here on earth. The relationship we formed, based on love, determination, and unwavering trust, is one I will cherish forever.

Cheryl's love for animals and all those who surrounded her radiated in her being. Her knowledge of veterinary medicine and innate ability to know her animal patients was remarkable. Bunny Boy and I owed her our deepest gratitude for helping to give him the long, full life that he had.

Bunny Boy taught me that unconditional love heals. He was a breath of fresh air that blew into my life, unknowingly, changing our family forever. Our indelible bond grew in sickness and in health. He was, in the end, my role model for how to conduct oneself with dignity—even when life throws you one difficult or humiliating curveball after another. He was my friend, my third child, my Bunny Boy.

This memoir is a work constructed from memory. It reflects the author's present recollections of experiences over time. Some names and identifying details have been changed to protect the privacy of the people involved.

Foreword

The first thing I learned about rabbit medicine after graduating vet school is that rabbits are born victims. They are nervous, skittish, defenseless creatures whose only hope is outrunning whatever is pursuing them. They evolved upon this planet as the perfect food source for most predators. They are difficult to treat medically as they often succumb to their fears and to pain. Anesthesia is riskier in rabbits than in other mammals. Frankly, they give up easier than most mammals. Not Bunny Boy.

Bunny Boy had the heart of a lion. He was anything but skittish. He was loved, and he loved back. He overcame medical problems that most rabbits die from within a year of the onset of their illness. He fought back regally and endured countless procedures. He had survived surgeries, medications, MRIs, CT scans, and two episodes of cardiac arrest. He was a rabbit unto his own. We warned his people time and time again that eventually the chronic infections would take their toll, told them countless times that he may not survive one more procedure. We tried to prepare them for the inevitable. Well, the inevitable did not come for eight years.

Bunny Boy was one of a kind. He cooperated when we needed him to. He allowed us to clean and dress his wounds. He allowed Nancy to hand-feed him when his teeth needed to be extracted due to chronic infections in his jaw. He was a kind, gentle soul who brought hope and happiness to all he touched. He surprised us and made us smile. He fought back when he shouldn't have had the strength. He had an impact on every person in the animal hospital. He has given us reason to believe that other rabbits can live with similar ailments. He has given us inspiration.

We all loved him and he will be missed.

—Cheryl Welch, VMD

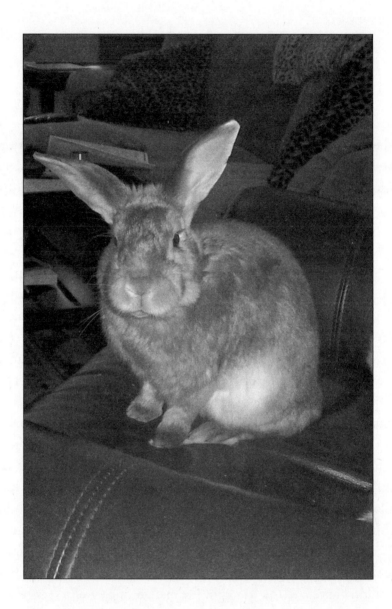

Introduction

When I was eight years old, my parents finally agreed to get us a dog. My little brother Tommy, who had been very sick from birth, had just received a clean bill of health. I think it was our parents' way of letting us know that the coast was clear that life could, at last, go on as normal.

I was four years old when Tommy, the youngest of five children in our Irish Catholic family, was born. The celebration began before Tommy even took his first breath. While our mother was in the hospital for three days, my father split his time between the hospital and our home, pulling out all the stops when it came to organizing festivities for the occasion. We dined on spam and cheese on a hard roll, drank Yoo-hoo, raised hell, and stayed up all night. Mom was a registered nurse who insisted on healthy meals and reasonable bed times, so the temporary free-for-all was like Christmas and New Year's and our birthdays all rolled up into one.

From the moment Tommy came home, with his jet-black hair tied with a yellow ribbon, we adored him. However, within months it became obvious that Tommy was not thriving the way he should have. By the time his first birthday came around, he had been rushed to the hospital by ambulance several times with serious breathing issues and convulsions. Before long, our baby brother was diagnosed with cystic fibrosis. The prognosis was poor, and the celebrations around our house ceased abruptly. Our newfound joy was replaced by a kind of anxious anticipation, dread of what was around the next hairpin turn on the roller coaster of our lives.

Months passed. Seasons came and went. Mom looked thin and worn out. Dad didn't smile quite as often. We took turns trying to keep Tommy comfortable and entertained. When he needed oxygen, we sat quietly with him, watching television or reading him a book. Tommy rarely complained when he couldn't come outside with us to play. His spirit was remarkable.

Then, one day, like an unexpected gift from above, things flip-flopped. After years of the same discouraging news, we got a reprieve. Newer, more comprehensive tests determined that my little brother did not have cystic fibrosis at all but rather acute asthma. Within months of proper treatment, Tommy began to flourish like any other four-year-old. Finally, he could come outside and play with the rest of us. I believe it was then that my parents decided the time was right to adopt the family's first pet. We could pick up where we had left off. It was the celebration of Tommy's rebirth.

We weren't a family with much disposable income. Raising five children on a nurse's and a machine foreman's salaries meant we had to watch every penny. So, we weren't exactly in the market for a pedigree pup. We needed a charity case, a lost pup who needed us as badly as we needed her. As luck would have it, a neighborhood family had just announced at Sunday mass that their dog, which was of no distinct lineage, had just given birth to five puppies. Fortune, it seemed, after years of scowling, had smiled upon us a second time in a week.

Our family meeting after church was nothing short of a summit of great minds and varied opinions on how to pick the perfect pup in the litter. We all had our various screening criteria, but our carefully calculated calibration theories went out the window the moment the puppies charged us, swarming across the plush green lawn like honeybees in search of the sweetest flower. The game was on. The score was even. There were five of them and five of us. One adorable puppy for each. But which one would we take home? It was impossible to choose.

Finally, the runt of the litter flopped down at my feet and looked up at me with loving, mournful eyes. She had silky blond fur, a black snout, and a tail that curled up like a donut. I loved her instantly.

"I think we should call her Flop," I said, knowing we had found our puppy. And somehow, the puppy knew it too. Flop looked up at me, as if to say, *Enough inspecting; I'm perfect. You know it as well as I do, so take me home already!* We all looked at each other; everyone else knew, too. Flop was our dog. No voting required. My oldest brother, Mike, carried Flop home in a large box. We laughed at how quickly we had picked the puppy's name, realizing we had deprived ourselves of a moment of family bickering at its finest. Our family had a brand-new member.

Having a puppy around the house was like extra gravy on your mashed potatoes. I was crazy about Flop, and I wasn't alone. We all loved her, and soon so did the whole neighborhood. Flop had a calm, nurturing temperament that fit in perfectly with our raucous group of seven. It was as if she had been custom created just for us. Flop would curl up in my armpit and rest her nose on my cheek, as my heart melted. She loved to ride in the car on family trips, tear around the little league field while my father coached, or follow me around on my bike. She memorized my brothers' paper routes, striking up friendships with anyone along the way, including the mayor. Our less-than-pedigree pup had become the town mascot.

Flop conquered us all with her instinctual understanding of what each of us needed at any given moment, and she always, without fail, delivered in full. When Flop was three years old, my father had his first massive heart attack. True to form, Flop sensed how much he needed her. During his long days home from work as he recovered, she never left his side. My dad and his faithful companion would walk to the mailbox together and then around the neighborhood. She would bring him the mail or just cozy up next to him on the sofa while he watched *All in the Family* or the news. Flop understood that what my dad needed most was somebody to keep him company.

One terrible summer afternoon, while she was delivering newspapers with my brothers, a truck hit Flop, killing her instantly. I felt like I had lost a part of my heart. I had loved her with my soul. I was afraid I would never stop crying. For weeks, my brothers barely spoke. Dad couldn't open the mail without tearing up. Mom left Flop's food and water bowl where they had always been for over a month. My sister, Carol, and I picked fresh flowers from our yard weekly and placed them on her small grave until the first frost set in. The mayor of our town was so upset at Flop's passing that he offered to buy us a new dog when we were ready. We were inconsolable.

During the nine years we were lucky enough to have Flop, she had become a beloved member of our family, as well as a member of just about every family in town. She taught me and everyone she came into contact with some of the most important lessons in life: that sometimes the unluckiest breaks in the world can turn out to be the luckiest, that the healing power of unconditional love is infinite, and that the simple act of being together and caring for each other through good times and bad are some of the universe's very best medicines.

From the day we lost Flop, I dreamed of her often and wondered if I would ever have another animal in my life whom I would love and who would love me as much. In true flip-flop fashion, it would take another streak of really bad luck to find out the answer to that question.

This is the story of our beloved family rabbit, Bunny Boy, who suffered more indignities than any rabbit ought to have (including spending the first part of his life saddled with the name Fluffett), but whose bravery and joie de vivre taught us more than a thing or two about how to live life to its fullest.

Chapter 1

We weren't old but we weren't young; we weren't rich but we weren't poor. We hadn't realized all of our dreams, but we'd seen more than a few come true and a few others dashed. We had come pretty far, but we still had some way to go. We were, in fact, right smack dab in the middle.

It was January 2001. My oldest child, Julie, was starting middle school, ready to jump into adolescence with both feet. Our accident-prone youngest, Chris, was about to make his first communion and had gone almost a whole year without needing stitches somewhere on his body—a new record. Ward, my husband, was in the middle of a merger that would quadruple the scale of his law practice. And I, at forty years of age, was in the middle of a remission from a mixed connective tissue disease and fibromyalgia, a remission long enough to let me hope that maybe it would last forever. Somehow, the Laracys had reached a place where life had come into perfect balance. And so, of course, I had to rock the boat.

It started with a simple conversation, as complicated things often do. It was a discussion my husband and I were both familiar with. We'd had it successfully twice before, so I saw no reason why anything should go differently this time. We had somewhat agreed from the start that we would have four kids. And while it was true that my illness had put things on hold, I was better now and didn't see why we shouldn't pick up right where we left off.

"Ward," I said, sitting down next to him by a roaring fire after the kids had finally gone to bed, "I want another baby, honey." Ward made a feeble attempt not to look shocked but failed miserably.

"Do you think that's wise with your health?" Ward's tone told me that this was purely a rhetorical question; to him, I must have been out of my mind to suggest such a thing after what I'd been through.

"I feel strong now," I said confidently, but Ward wasn't buying it.

"Nance, I don't think it's a good idea," he said. I was startled at the resolution in his voice. He meant business. I suddenly felt my jaw set in the way it does when the iron will I inherited from my Irish mother starts to make itself known.

"Ward, you can't just tell me no more babies. That would be like me saying to you that you can't practice law any more. I'm a mom. I'm a nurturer. This is what I love to do. You can't just say no like that."

"No, Nancy. We have enough on our plate." Ward was sympathetic but firm. "It's just too much, for all of us. Let's enjoy what we have."

And that's when I started to get mad.

Of course, I knew Ward was probably right. I had been in remission for a while, but there was no guarantee that it would last. My life was a roller coaster—it always had been, a series of unexpected twists and plunges since I was young. I could never be completely sure what was around the next bend.

When I was twenty-two, my dad died suddenly of a heart attack on his fifty-eighth birthday. Nothing could have prepared me for the sudden and profound loss of my father. Life seemed to crumble in front of me. My unwavering faith encountered a bump in the road. My emotions fluctuated from shock to grief to anger, and back to shock. The tears gushed like a mountain stream after a winter thaw, raging their way from the peak to the valley below, and I began to reach out to God in a way I never had before, in order to deal with the strength of the current. While I had shared with Dad a piece of his birthday cake earlier that fateful evening, I was not with him when he died.

A week after he left us, Dad appeared to me while I was sitting at my desk in my bedroom. He and two white angels slowly glided toward me like fog coming over the mountain. I recall my body freezing, and I felt damp and cold.

He spoke to me softly. "Everything is going to be okay. I am fine now."

How could Dad possibly think everything was going to be fine? I had lost my rock. I wanted to speak to him, but no words came to my shivering lips. My father's blue eyes seemed brighter than I remembered. They were filled with joy—not the sorrow or fear I had seen so many times when he was in the hospital with his first heart attacks. Suddenly, warmth swept through me as my father lightly placed his arms around my shoulders. I felt as if I had been wrapped in a large cape made of cotton candy. It was a miraculous, spiritual moment I will never forget, a pivotal point in my life. It was then that I established my own adult relationship with God.

The months and years that followed my father's death were bittersweet. I missed his stability and good advice, but most of all his love. I moved forward with my studies, later meeting the challenges of an exciting career in executive recruiting. I met my first love, Ward; and when he finished law school, we married. Walking down the aisle on my brother Tommy's arm to meet my future husband, I glanced up toward the stained glass windows in the church I considered my home and felt my father's presence, watching over me from above.

More years than I would like to admit sped by, and suddenly I found myself as a stay-at-home mother with a beautiful child. During the third trimester of my fourth pregnancy (I had had two back-to-back miscarriages), we sold our first home, a sixties-style lake house forty minutes outside of New York City, and bought a larger house with oodles of character in an affluent neighborhood in northern New Jersey. I gave birth to our second bundle of joy by Caesarean section. With a six-week-old baby in one arm and a three-year-old toddler in the other, I packed endless boxes and moved into our Georgian side-door colonial. The years that followed were a blur.

Then, while I was hurtling through life full throttle, harsh reality stopped me dead in my tracks. A virus—parvovirus B19—struck when I was thirty-seven years old and wreaked havoc on my body for over a year, specifically my immune system, weakening it and causing a "glitch" in its normal operations. I developed a connective tissue disease—and then fibromyalgia about a year later. There was no cure for either disease.

My connective tissue disease essentially meant that my body had not yet decided what I had—lupus or rheumatoid arthritis. Fibromyalgia, once thought to be rheumatism of the muscles, at least when I was first diagnosed, is now thought to be a disease of the central nervous system where the nerves in your body misfire. It is believed to be caused by a chronic infection, like the one I had, or a physical injury, emotional trauma, or chronic stress. In my case, parvovirus B19 was the etiological agent for my fibromyalgia.

In a strange way, I felt grateful that I never had to live with the stigma often associated with fibromyalgia. In my case, I fell sick so acutely and quickly from parvovirus B19 that, within a week of contracting the virus, I went from managing two children and a household to being nearly crippled with arthritis in all my joints and plagued with high fevers. In contrast to my very visible pain, most fibromyalgia patients typically develop pain slowly over the years from emotional stress or multiple traumas. As a result, they often find themselves having to answer to other people's skepticism about their pain—is it all real? Sadly, you cannot always see the pain associated with fibromyalgia, save for extreme cases where patients finds themselves bedridden. Patients often hear the words, "But you look fine," despite the agony they may feel. The invisible nature of fibromyalgia can be emotionally devastating.

My life, and my family's, was turned upside down. The next few years were spent enduring one medical treatment after another. Whether mainstream or holistic, whatever I thought might possibly help, I tried. My extended Buchalski family helped out with household chores, food shopping, and meal preparation while I reserved what little energy I had for my two children and husband, the primary reasons why I woke up most mornings with the will to continue.

There were many times, however, when I wanted to give up. The pain ravaged my entire body. In the early years, there were times when I could barely touch the skin on my chest and extremities due to the burning and extreme sensitivity. The fatigue was crushing—like someone had unplugged my energy source. I reached for my faith once again to guide me through the difficult days, fully expecting to wake up from the nightmare. But it seemed like I never would. With time, the dream simply faded into the distance, tucked in the back of my mind, reminding me of my limits.

After what felt like an eternity, I began to experience periods of relative wellness followed by periodic setbacks. I continued to raise my children under difficult circumstances, letting the nonessential things slip by. I knew the delivery people from the pharmacy, supermarket, and takeout restaurants by their first names. Sunday mass, family gatherings, holiday events, and birthday parties got top priority. Most fibromyalgia patients keep fighting to maintain some sense of normalcy in their lives by hiding their pain and pushing through it—and that was exactly what I did. Meanwhile, I focused intensely on regaining my health by incorporating a regular routine of physical therapy, chiropractic treatment, and a much healthier diet.

Now, at age forty, I felt better, stronger, and ready to think about having another baby before it was too late. I had earned it. I had worked hard to put myself in a place where I could build a larger family like I had always wanted. But once again, my illness and now my husband were reminding me that I had my limits.

This made me mad—at Ward and at the whole world. I was angry that I had gotten sick. I was angry that I might have to give up my lifelong dream of having four children. And, just like every other time I'd gone head to head with my diseases, I was determined to push the envelope and demand the most out of life, no matter what the chronic pain had to say about it. I didn't know what was going to happen, but I knew I wasn't going to give up.

And then, something did happen. At 9 p.m. on the evening of our conversation, it started to snow, continuing throughout the night. The firehouse sirens had gone off, signaling no school. The airwaves were filled with ominous warnings not to travel unless absolutely necessary. But I felt comforted by the storm. In my world, the worst had already happened, which I have learned can be very liberating. Everything is less frightening somehow when the other shoe has already dropped.

● ● ●

The next morning, I peered out the window of our cozy Georgian colonial, small by Franklin Lakes standards but lovable and warm, and to me, who had grown up in a small Cape Cod with four siblings, practically palatial. Our neighborhood was blanketed in pristine winter white. The snowflakes were large, fluffy, and relentless. The wind had already blown the snow into great drifts, creating a transformed mystical landscape in our backyard. The lanterns on the porch were translucent, covered in thick snow with just a hint of light shining through.

"Snow day! Snow day!" my kids shouted at the top of their lungs, rushing into the kitchen. They had slept with their pajamas inside out the night before, a superstition which was supposed to guarantee them a snow day. They giggled gleefully and gave each other a high five, overjoyed that their brand of special magic had worked like a charm.

I was as excited as my children to have a snow day. I love winter. The season was the backdrop for some of my fondest memories, and it offered many opportunities for themed baking and family gatherings, both passions of mine. I loved most winter sports, or at least I did until I got sick. But today was a good day, and I felt like I could do anything in the world if I wanted to badly enough. I was in the mood for an adventure. And the kids and I had a whole day to figure out what it would be.

I walked to the fridge and pulled out the Pillsbury Cinnamon Rolls—a snow day tradition passed on from my mother, who taught me most of what I know about making a moment feel special. My mother was strong, independent, feisty, and as resourceful as they come; but she was also extremely sentimental and she had a great sense of playfulness. As a nurse who cared for the elderly, she somehow raised five children while being the sole caretaker for my chronically ill Dad and little brother. Yet she always found time to lend a hand to anybody in our neighborhood who needed help. Both of my parents had an amazing way of keeping us together as a family. Whether it was going to Goody's, the first fast food burger joint in our town, or piling all of us into one hotel room so we could afford a weekend family getaway, we always made the most of what we had. And now, no matter how many obstacles we had to face, my family, too, always found a way to make the best of things.

Julie and Chris settled in the family room on separate sofas, munching on their cinnamon buns. Julie was wrapped in her favorite leopard blanket, Chris in his prized cheetah print. The sun made a brief appearance, bursting through the clouds to show a brilliant and blue sky, making the trees sparkle like they had been spray-painted with white glitter. I started daydreaming about Julie and Chris as babies in snowsuits, pulled along by Ward on their flexible flyer up the little hill so they could sled down again, their cheeks rosy and noses running from the cold. Where had the time gone?

I had gotten very good at daydreaming over the last few years—because I'd had to. Taking myself away in my mind was sometimes the only way for me to cope with the pain. Listen, pain happens. Shins get kicked, heads get bumped, bones get broken, and skin gets burned. People curse or sometimes cry. They catch their breath. The bone gets set and the wound heals. Eventually, pain subsides. That's the simple kind of pain—it may hurt a lot, but it plays fair.

Chronic pain, on the other hand, is unrelenting, unpredictable, and unfair. It can bully with moods, jobs, and relationships, and it affected my ability to be a mom and a wife. But the day I was diagnosed with a connective tissue disease and fibromyalgia, I decided that there's pain, and then there's your *reaction* to pain. That part was up to me, and I was fighting back with everything I had. I wasn't going to let pain control my life or my family's.

Some days, the throbbing neck and back pain was all-consuming. After one trip to the emergency room from bad side effects, I tossed all my pain medications into the garbage and started going to a chiropractor. I scheduled weekly massages to help relieve the widespread muscle pain. At times, it felt like a thousand knives piecing my entire body. The weight of a light blanket was so painful that I would sleep uncovered. I walked on an underwater treadmill at physical therapy to remove stress from the painful joints while my muscles strengthened. I cringed when small jolts of electricity shot through my body at the acupuncturist. I forced my husband to sleep with me on a magnetic mattress designed to alleviate pain. I saw a psychologist who warned, "You might never be the old you again; you may get depressed and develop anxiety." His words only made me that much more determined to beat the pain. People would say, "Just accept it and give into it." But I couldn't. If I had accepted my fate, there wouldn't have been days like today.

By mid-morning, our backyard was full of neighborhood children and enormous inflatable snow tubes, all tangled up together like living, giggling sculptures. We always had a lot of traffic at our house, which I enjoyed. My childhood house was always packed with kids and animals and laughter and love. I adored the chaos—to me, it felt like home. Once the sun began to set, everybody came in for one last round of hot chocolate and delicious treats that I had made. Then they wandered out into the winter wonderland with full bellies and pink cheeks.

"Mom! Sunny needs crickets." Chris came bouncing down the stairs with his usual reckless abandon that made me think he was about to go sailing over the railing and land on his head at any moment. It had happened before. Sunny was our Australian bearded dragon who had a seemingly bottomless appetite for crickets and romaine lettuce. Chris had wanted a puppy, but Ward was allergic, so he was making the best of things.

"The lettuce is gone, too. Can we go to Scuffy's?" Chris grinned mischievously. He knew that I knew that the crickets were just a handy excuse to visit his beloved pet store. Well, this was a family emergency. Venturing out into the snow against the advice of local officials had become unavoidable. So we dug out the family vehicle and headed off to the pet store without giving the swirling Snowmageddon a second thought.

Scuffy's Pet Store, remarkably, was open, despite the fact that the mall parking lot looked like a frigid steppe straight out of *Dr. Zhivago*. We parked next to buried SUVs that would clearly not be seeing the light of day until the great thaw arrived. It really was an epic blizzard. What were we thinking coming out into this? But I was not afraid of much of anything those days. And somehow, because of that, we seemed to be able to run where angels feared to tread and get to the other side in one piece.

Julie and Chris rushed into the store, nearly banging headfirst into the manager, Stacey, who was holding an adorable white ball of fluff.

"Chris, this is a Bijon," Stacey said to my son, who looked skeptical. "He's a dog your father won't be allergic to." Everyone knew that Chris had wanted a puppy almost as bad as I wanted another baby, but I could see that this diminutive dog wasn't measuring up to the scale of his puppy fantasies.

"That's not a dog," Chris muttered, with the royal disdain only a nine-year-old boy can summon. I smiled and petted the puppy apologetically.

"Sorry, little guy. I think Chris has something more like a big chocolate Labrador in mind." I went about my usual business, ordering forty live crickets in a cup. The things we do for love.

Julie and Chris made their rounds among the cages stocked with puppies, kittens, turtles, and hamsters. Then, they stopped short.

"Mom! Come look!" I shuffled over to oblige them. At that moment, I had not realized that what I would find in the pen at their feet was about to change our lives forever. I looked down.

It was a litter of bunnies. Some were sleeping, curled up together like fuzzy spoons. Others kicked up their hind legs playfully and nibbled on each other's ears. We all focused in on one bunny who was off on her own. She looked like a miniature version of the Easter Bunny, and her fur was the color of cinnamon sprinkled on snow.

"She's a dwarf. A red satin," said Loretta, another employee at the store who was also our Australian bearded dragon expert. She lifted the tiny bunny out of the sweet pool of fur on the floor and handed her to me. Despite the frigid theme of the day, something in me began to melt. She wasn't much bigger than a softball. She sat looking at us, trembling. Her pink nose twittered, her oversized ears twitched. There was such a sense of mystery emanating from this tiny, warm ball of fur. It was as if I could somehow sense, on a level that is beyond knowing, everything that we would come to mean to each other in the years ahead.

Of course, I paid no further attention to this at the time. All I knew was that she was irresistible and felt wonderful in my arms.

"It's a kit. That's what you call a baby bunny," Loretta explained, winking at me and tickling the bunny's nose with her finger. "They can make wonderful house pets," she added slyly.

"She's so sweet," I said, stroking the indescribably soft spot behind her ears. Julie and Chris looked at me with the same mournful eyes as the bunny. Apparently, I wasn't the only pushover in the room.

"We'll take her!" I blurted out suddenly. To this day, I'm not exactly sure what came over me. The kids' jaws dropped to the floor.

"Really, Mom?" said Julie, giving me her familiar side-eye. With a daughter who was just entering the eye-rolling, lip-curling brink of adolescence, I had already come to know that look well. "Don't you think Dad will be mad?"

"He might," I said, feeling the tickle of a canary feather at the corner of my lips. In the wake of our conversation the night before, I had decided to make this bunny my Waterloo. There was no turning back now.

We let Loretta lead us around the store while we grabbed supplies off of the shelves with reckless abandon, accumulating every known bunny accessory in the industrialized world. The kids were hesitant at first with my unfamiliar burst of bunny rebellion, but they joined in soon enough once we chanced upon the McMansion-sized cage that would be the rabbit's new home.

I rarely, if ever, did anything on the home front that Ward and I hadn't discussed and agreed to beforehand, especially when it came to new family members. As a lawyer, Ward believed in due process, and generally I followed it to the letter. Lately though—perhaps because of my conversation with him or my illness, or because my kids were getting older and learning to make their own decisions—it seemed like so much of my life involved negotiation, compromise, concessions, and constant procedural delays about the simplest things that could be avoided.

Today, I just wanted to do something spontaneous. I wanted, for once, to do something just because I *wanted* to. The moment I set eyes on her, I knew I needed this bunny. And somehow, I also knew, in the way that you do, that the bunny needed me.

We traipsed back out into the snow and headed for home with crickets for Sunny and our humongous cage; enough hay, food, and toys for an entire litter of bunnies; a few books on how to care for rabbits; and, of course, our new bunny. Now I just had to figure out how to tell my husband that he had become the proud new father of an eight-week-old red satin kit—someone who was about to take center stage in our lives and change everything.

Chapter 2

Ward was waiting in the kitchen when we walked in from the garage. "We just had a little cabin fever and went to the pet store," I had told him earlier when he called my cell phone, wondering where his family could possibly be during this awful snowstorm. "I'll be home in five minutes, honey," I continued happily, as if driving in a blizzard was something any mother would do when her kids got bored. "We have a surprise."

I dragged the cage in. "She'll be perfect right here, kids," I said, pointing to a corner near the closet, as if I had just bought a piece of furniture instead of a pet.

"You bought the kids a rabbit without at least asking me, Nance?"

"I did," I replied, with haughtiness that surprised even me.

The dead silence was awkward while we both carefully prepared our responses. Five seconds seemed like an eternity. Catching me off guard, Ward skipped what I thought might be a rigorous interrogation and cut to the chase.

"What if I am allergic to her?"

Before he could say another word, Chris came to my rescue and plopped the tiny ball of fur in his father's arms.

"Look how cute she is, Dad!"

Ward fidgeted awkwardly, trying to make the baby bunny comfortable on his chest. She seemed swallowed up in his large arms. Then, as if the gods were on my side, she made a sharp twist with her body and was suddenly face to face with Ward. Ever so sweetly, she started nibbling on his tie, almost sensing that this big guy was the one she needed to win over.

"She *is* kinda cute." Ward rubbed the bunny's head softly with his knuckles. Discreetly, Chris gave me the thumbs up, and I could feel some of the stress in my shoulders disappear as the bunny's body began to relax against Ward's chest. I watched for any signs of a runny nose or hives appearing on Ward's neck, which happened almost immediately when he was near a cat or dog.

"She's Julie's birthday present," Chris added, winking at Julie. Julie's birthday was coming up in March, and the kids and I had agreed on the ride home that it was the perfect reason for buying a bunny.

Within minutes, we were all in the family room, watching the little bunny frolic in her new surroundings. Ward sat at his desk, clutching a bottle of Benadryl and shaking his head periodically in disbelief. The bunny was no bigger than the palm of your hand. Her pure white belly and tail resembled soft balls of cotton. Her features were delicate except for her tall ears, which were disproportionate to her small size. Then, she did the cutest thing. All two pounds of fluff flipped in the air, as though she had springs on her tiny feet, as she twisted her body. This, we later learned, is called *binkying* or *popcorning*, which is a bunny's sign of playfulness and their unique way of communicating, "I am so happy."

"How big will she get?" Ward asked, cracking a smile. Of course, I knew he was referring to the McMansion-size cage.

"The cage was Chris's idea," said Julie helpfully.

While the kids and I sat on the floor, the bunny continued to scamper around the furniture, sniffing everything with her head down like a pig searching for truffles. Julie and Chris squealed delightfully as she hopped around their legs, brushing her fluffy tail up against their feet. When her twittering nose and whiskers tickled my toes, I thought I would burst with excitement. Suddenly, it didn't seem to matter how painful every muscle in my body felt as I sat cross-legged on the floor. As Julie and Chris smothered their new bunny with kisses, warmth filled my heart as I watched their unbridled affection toward our new family member. I couldn't remember a happier moment in our family in a long time.

We mulled over a few bunny names, but our creativity was seriously lacking. Thankfully, bedtime became imminent and we would decide later. And thanks to the luck of the bunny, perhaps, Ward didn't need to take any Benadryl. I painstakingly followed the directions for "cage set-up," and grabbed one of my old pink baby blankets from the linen closet and draped it over the bunny's cage with the tender love of a mother. "Goodnight little one," I whispered.

That night in bed, visions of the kit clinging to her siblings kept me from sleeping. Imaginary nocturnal cries haunted me. At midnight, I took my first trip down the stairs to check on the bunny. I found her cowering in the corner of the cage, probably afraid of the dark. So we cuddled for a bit before I went back up to bed. My two o' clock sojourn down to the kitchen was noticeably more difficult as the nighttime stiffness and pain had taken over my body. Tickled pink to see our baby bunny, we cuddled again for about a half hour, during which she peed on my soft bathrobe. By three o'clock, she was restless and had no interest in snuggling. She wriggled with verve and energy while I struggled to keep my eyes open. When I let her down on the living room rug, she tore across the room like she had just escaped from prison. I suppose she had. She gnawed at the white moldings, chewed the skirt to the sofa, and nibbled the shoes I had left under the coffee table—all while leaving a trail of poop along her path of destruction, little brown balls. But I didn't care. She was so adorable. She popped onto my lap for a split second and then returned to her next task on hand—chinning everything and marking her territory.

When I could barely keep my eyes open any longer, I tried putting her in the cage but she swung her front and back legs wildly as if she were about to fly and fell headfirst into her pile of hay. In an instant she rolled over and landed on all fours with a small thud. Then she looked up at me adoringly. As I leaned down, she grabbed the rungs of the cage with her tiny front paws and stuck her nose through, staring at me with pleading eyes. Clearly, she didn't want to be locked up, alone without her siblings. I curled up on the floor next to her cage, and she nuzzled her soft face against my hand. My heart started to flutter.

"Do you miss your siblings?" I asked softly. "This is your new home now."

I started to hum, and her head dropped down and her back paws relaxed beneath her body. She tapped my nose gently with her left paw and stared at me intently. No whining. No barking. But guilt struck a motherly chord, and for the next half hour I lay on the hard tile floor next to her cage, talking to her and stroking her soft fur. I didn't care that my body ached. Luckily, for the bunny's sake, waking up half a dozen times during the night was nothing out of the ordinary for me. Insomnia was just one of the many other frustrating symptoms of fibromyalgia that I had learned to live with. After about an hour of lying in such an uncomfortable position, I decided I had better get some sleep before my chronic pain worsened.

Regretfully, I whispered my final goodnight. The last image I saw was her tiny pink nose poking out from under the blanket.

I woke up a few hours later to the usual "Good morning, egg," Ward's pet phrase for me since the early days of our marriage. It was my barometer for how things were going; it was all about the tone. Today's was monotone.

I slipped out of bed and walked downstairs, smiling mischievously. My mind wandered to our kit—her ginger-colored fur and tiny paws. Drifts of snow were piled up along the balusters lining the colonial-style deck and the snow blowing off the roof of the storage shed was glitterlike. Julie and Chris were hovering over the bunny's cage. Chris had that early morning look—tussled hair and dried crusty sleep in the corner of his eyes. Julie sported her Hello Kitty pajamas and feline slippers. They both looked irresistibly adorable—as did our new bunny.

She was balancing a piece of hay between her tall ears while she nibbled on another—like an act from a circus. Her mouth shimmied from side to side as her two sets of top molars aligned themselves with the single set of molars on the bottom. But her cage was anything but cute. It looked like a cyclone had hit it. Hay and food pellets were scattered everywhere, and her toys were haphazardly piled up in the corner. She must have thrown a tantrum after I went up to bed.

We would quickly learn that a rabbit's days are framed by the rising and setting of the sun. Crepuscular animals are most active at dawn and dusk, as well as awake during the nighttime between. It was clear that the bunny had not slept at all.

Chris no sooner had let the rabbit out of her cage when Julie screamed, "She's my bunny!" I stood on the sidelines, hoping to remain uninvolved. Unexpectedly, Chris made the hand-off of our new prized possession to Julie ever so gently and without much fuss. The bunny started squirming wildly in Julie's arms.

"Rabbits are skittish animals," I said to the kids, quoting Loretta from Scuffy's, while praying silently that Julie would not drop the bunny. "You need to spend time with them on the floor where they feel most comfortable—on all fours."

They lowered themselves to the ground slowly, huddled around the bunny as if they wanted to discuss something I shouldn't hear.

"You need to earn a bunny's trust slowly," I continued. "It doesn't come naturally to them. They are very different than dogs or cats." I had absorbed more of Loretta's CliffsNotes on how to raise a house rabbit than I'd thought while I stood in the store, completely mesmerized by the magical bunny with the coal-colored eyes.

When the kids broke their huddle, Julie let the bunny loose from her grasp. Surprisingly, the rabbit didn't move. I crouched down, tapped her super-soft backside playfully, and perched my head on Julie's shoulder. After a few seconds, the baby bunny reached her front paws out on the hard tile tentatively, one at a time, as if testing the temperature of the ocean.

"She's being cautious because bunnies don't like hard surfaces," Chris explained, repeating another fun fact we had learned at the pet store.

Despite the hardness of the tile, once our kit got her bearings, she began racing in and out around the legs of the table and chairs like she was running through a maze. She popped up sharply numerous times, facing different directions—the behavior that is called *binkying* or *pop-corning*—and then scurried down the hallway toward the bathroom, sniffing the molding along the way. She charged forward and slid across the marble floor, and then crashed into the wall behind the toilet. Her tiny body sunk to the floor like it had been deflated. She started shaking like a leaf, her tall ears flopped down toward her backside. Her nose was twittering in fast motion.

Loretta's words flashed through my mind. "They can easily injure their backs! Bunnies are prone to heart attacks if they are frightened!"

I whisked the bunny up and cuddled her on my chest beneath my bathrobe. I could feel my heart pounding along with hers as she remained frightfully still.

"Is she hurt, Mom?" Julie asked anxiously. I moved the bunny's limbs slowly—checking for fractures—and palpated her small body for punctured organs. I inspected the vertebrae on her spine like a skilled orthopedic surgeon. In an attempt to ward off hysteria from the kids, I responded, "I think she's fine." Secretly, I worried that the bunny would be scarred for life. In less than eighteen hours, she had been taken away from her siblings and forced to navigate her way around hard floors, and now she had had her first brush with disaster.

But any semblance of empathy disappeared from Julie's demeanor when the bunny, seemingly making a miraculous recovery, started wriggling to get free. Julie plucked the bunny out of my arms and put her back on the floor. Our kit circled the table and chairs with more vim and vigor, and then she flipped her body with a twist and headed back toward the bathroom. She stopped dead in her tracks as she approached the marble tile, and then swung her hind legs up and turned back toward us.

"We have a baby Einstein," I exclaimed, certain I had just seen the first glimpse of our new family member's intelligence.

"Don't get carried away, Mom," replied Chris. "Rabbits aren't that smart."

I knew I would have to prove Chris wrong.

Ward walked down the stairs hurriedly, already late for a meeting, and asked what all the commotion was, as if he had forgotten I'd brought home a bunny the night before. He looked handsome in his gray tailored suit, white shirt, and pink paisley tie.

"We have a third baby Einstein," I said, beaming like a proud parent. "I picked the pedigree of the herd."

He smiled but barely engaged me, except to remind me that it was Julie who actually shared Albert Einstein's birthday, March 14.

We all sensed his coolness as he walked briskly out the door. The kids looked at me quizzically.

"No worries," I said. "He'll come around."

Chapter 3

"*Usted compró un conejo?*" Tina asked.

You bought a bunny?

"*Sí, sí.* I did," I said.

I pulled away from the bus stop where I picked up Tina, the loving and caring woman who helped us keep some semblance of order in our home after we reluctantly accepted the realization that I wasn't going to return to my "type A on steroids" self any time soon. Tina, a native of Honduras, had came to the United States on a work visa and was granted permanent residence by President Clinton after the devastating Hurricane Mitch struck in 1998. She lived with us part-time and had become part of our family. A godsend in every way, we had all grown to love her.

Tina had dark brown hair and a solid build with broad shoulders, and she walked with a slight limp due to a childhood hip injury. Her skin was slightly weathered from years of tropical sun, and her rough hands were a product of farming and domestic work. She had a smile that seemed to be etched permanently on her round face and a gentleness and a warmth that radiated from her being. She was quite social, a necessary attribute to fit in with my incredibly not-so-shy family. She also had a great sense of humor. I thoroughly enjoyed conversing with her in Spanish rather than in English, which drove my family crazy. They were never quite sure what I was saying about them! (Though it didn't take Ward long to figure out that "*muy mal hombre*" was not a compliment.)

Tina and I were deeply engrossed in Baby Einstein details when I spotted red flashing lights coming up behind me in my rearview mirror.

I pulled over onto the snow-covered shoulder of the road and waited for the officer.

"License and registration, please." He said, very businesslike. I apologized for speeding and blamed my infraction on the excitement over buying a bunny. There was a stray bag of hay on the backseat in plain sight. Tina tried to hide her shock at my ridiculous admission and muttered under her breath, "*Loco en la cabeza.*" I thought I saw the hint of a chuckle on the policeman's face as he walked back to his vehicle.

When he returned, he was holding a picture of a black-and-white lop-eared bunny in his hand, not a ticket.

"His name is Oreo," he said, with a silly grin. "I keep his picture in my wallet along with my children's."

Oreo was the runt of a litter who had been bred in South Jersey. "Lop-eared bunnies are very smart," he remarked, radiating with pride.

It seems we're all alike when it comes to bragging about our children and our pets.

He stood there on the side of the road for about ten minutes, giving me helpful tips on keeping a bunny indoors as though he knew as much about rearing a bunny as he did the law. Finally, he extended his hand to shake mine.

"Have a great day and enjoy your new bunny. She will win your heart!"

I drove home, winding around the snow-covered reservoir, thinking, *What were the chances of being pulled over by a police officer who had a pet bunny?*

I made my way through our vastly wooded, picturesque suburban town of Franklin Lakes, nestled just twenty-two miles outside of the metropolis of Manhattan. We had the luxury of living out in the country while still being part of the hustle and bustle of a big city, accessible in half an hour, depending on traffic. Named after Benjamin Franklin's grandson, our town had ten thousand residents and boasted top-notch schools and a keen sense of community. As I drove, the sun reflected off the snowcapped trees, nearly blinding me. Heavy snow-covered branches had formed a beautiful white canopy over the streets. Squirrels were scurrying across the wires, knocking off clumps of snow that formed a mist of white when they landed on my windshield with a thump.

When I pulled into the driveway, I noticed a mother and two baby deer munching on the barely visible tips of the holly bushes at the top of the hill in our backyard. I instantly envisioned our kit with her mother and siblings.

When Tina and I walked into the kitchen, we found the baby bunny plumping like a hen in the corner of her cage. She had kicked up a pile of litter, forming almost a pillow for herself. She made the cutest yawn when she saw me; her tiny front teeth reminded me of Chiclets. The kit stretched her soft body forward slowly, and then she lunged unexpectedly toward her water bottle and started lapping at the ball on the bottom of the spout with her head sideways, eyeing me. I waited patiently while she quenched her thirst. Then I scooped her up, barely able to wait another moment to cuddle with her. I kissed the side of her sweet face. She smelled like the fragrant pine shavings of her litter. She was light as a feather.

As she nuzzled her damp nose against mine, shivers went down my spine. I looked endearingly into her eyes, then outside the house at the remnants of the snowstorm. The icicles that hung from the gutters above the kitchen windows were melting from the warmth of the sun, creating small crevices in the snow beneath them. My heart, too, was melting. The bunny's whiskers tickled my neck. She was simply enchanting. I caressed her tall ears and could feel her body slowly relax against my cashmere sweater. Within minutes, my body had also begun to relax in tandem, and I noticed that my muscles suddenly didn't seem quite so sore. For me, my daily grind of getting up in the morning and performing simple tasks such as reaching for the coffee pot or opening the refrigerator for the cream increased my muscle pain. Opening the car door, climbing in, and turning my body to back up the car were difficult chores that pulled on my sore muscles. But today, my muscles seemed to feel a little different.

I let out a sigh of contentment. Tina, a mother herself, recognized the look. "You really did want another baby, didn't you?"

If I had only known what the bunny and I would come to mean to each other in the coming years.

Chapter 4

The packed yellow school bus pulled up at 3:15 p.m. Within minutes, the house was under siege. Backpacks flew and snow gear formed a pile in the foyer, left to melt on the floor.

It was the bunny's debut. The neighborhood children ran into the kitchen and swarmed the bunny's cage while Chris opened the front latch. Without a moment's hesitation, the baby bunny raced out and ran headfirst into a wall of feet. She backed up and binkied, switching directions three times, igniting gleeful sounds, then turned abruptly and started nibbling the masses of toes. When she got bored, she scampered off toward the dining room, blissful and without a care in the world. Relying on my own reflexes, I flew after our pint-sized lagomorph, the children racing behind me. But the bunny was faster. She slipped through my hands and bolted to the tea-dyed green and burgundy Persian carpet like a true prey animal, where she started nibbling the fringe on the rug so fast that, within seconds, an inch was missing. Her tiny mouth swished from side to side like she was rinsing her mouth with Listerine on high speed.

"Not the fringe!" I shrieked, whisking her up in my arms.

She looked up at me with her adorable eyes, as if to say, "Is there a problem? You thought I was cute last night when I was nibbling."

Chris clearly had an agenda for the day. He quickly asked if they could bring the bunny up to the family room, which doubled as a playroom. I hesitated, not sure I was ready to leave our bunny in the hands of such a raucous group. I looked at the missing fringe from the rug. "Sure," I said.

While I had never considered myself an overprotective mother, I felt a compelling need to make sure the bunny stayed safe, but I didn't want to be too overbearing. I assembled a tray of snacks and brought them up to the children. Then, to bide my time, I dusted the bookcases and coffee tables downstairs, replaced a few light bulbs, and tightened loose knobs on the cabinet doors. Then I went back up to the playroom and ran my stand-up seven-pound Dirt Devil Lite vacuum cleaner at the far end where some soil had spilled over from one of the plants. I made a mental note to get rid of the plants. Light housekeeping was about all I could manage without dramatically changing my pain level from tolerable to *bad*.

"Mom, bunnies hate loud noises!" Julie screeched, as the bunny appeared out of nowhere and hopped onto the head of the vacuum. Before I could hit the *off* button, our kit had started nibbling the plastic handle—curious rather than terrified. The kids quickly formed a circle around me, laughing heartily at the scene. The bunny showed no signs of stress from the noise of the vacuum or the chaos from the children.

"Mom, pleeeease, we want our privacy," Chris pleaded in between laughter.

Reluctantly, I retreated to the kitchen, dragging one of the chairs over toward the stairway so I could hear them better. When I felt satisfied that things were going smoothly, I started a simple dinner—stuffed peppers. We all loved stuffed peppers, except for Ward. We knew the story by heart—his mother used to stuff peppers with rice as an economy meal when his father was out of work and they had no money to buy meat.

"Sometimes, we ate just the peppers without any filling," he'd say for the umpteenth time. By that point, we were usually rolling our eyes and raising our hands as if to say, *enough*. "When we were desperate, she would just put a picture of a pepper on our plate," he'd finish, ignoring our pleas for him to stop.

I returned to the playroom an hour later to check on the bunny. I looked around for any possible infractions, specifically little brown balls or chewed items. There were none—yet. Our kit was playing among the

children, seemingly comfortable in her new home as they tickled and petted her endlessly. She plopped into a wicker basket and started nibbling
on one of Julie's Beanie Baby magazines.

"No no, sweetie," said Julie softly as she shooed the kit out of the
basket. "Not my magazines."

I barely recognized the sweet tone. Julie had recently morphed into
a tween—the difficult stage that prepares you for a worse stage that's yet
to come. Chris had taken Julie's personality change in stride, unlike me,
who took it personally.

In a nanosecond, the bunny regrouped and charged the basket, chewing the wicker with a frenetic pace. I swooped in and pried open her
mouth to find that a small piece of wicker had already made it past her
razor-sharp teeth. I was sure it would have made its way down her throat
to cause a blockage in her intestines. It was our second near-miss. Bunnies
have a one-way esophagus, and the unusual strength of their sphincter
muscle prevents them from throwing up hairballs or dangerous items or
substances. There would be no syrup of ipecac to help with these kinds
of emergencies.

I began to fret as I looked around the room at the dozens of wires
coming from the computer, the television, and the Nintendo 64. My eyes
moved to the kids' textbooks and a few stray sneakers. Chris must have
read my mind.

"The bunny better not chew my Nintendo wires or my headphones,"
he warned.

"We need to name the bunny," I said suddenly. I had already anticipated that naming our kit would set into motion a major squabble
between Julie and Chris and me, and secretly I hoped that their friends
might come up with more innovative names to choose from. I reached
into my pants pocket and took out a list of possible names I had carefully prepared while they were at school. In bright red letters, I'd written
down half a dozen adjectives that I thought described her fur exquisitely:
Caramel, Buttercup, Sandy, Creamsicle, Velvet, Ginger, and Satin. At the
bottom, written in black letters, were the bunny-sounding names that I
loathed: Snowball, Thumper, Fluffy, and Flopsy. Before I could suggest

a single name, Julie and Chris blurted out, "We like Fluffett, Mom. We already decided on the bunny's name."

I stood for a moment, speechless, not sure what bothered me more: the name or my lack of input. Sadly, I looked at my list.

"Fluffett?" I asked, desperately trying to hide my disappointment but failing miserably. *God, it's so pedestrian*, I thought. None of the other children offered a single name; they were strangely quiet. "What about Ginger, like in Ginger Rogers?" I asked in a pleading tone. "She was a famous movie star."

"We never heard of her, Mom."

Of course they hadn't.

"And it has cache. Fluffett is so ordinary," I pleaded. I wanted to say, "I hate Fluffett!"

"But we like Fluffett," they said firmly.

I foolishly looked toward their friends for help, but the children were now all nodding their heads in agreement. "It's the perfect bunny name, Mrs. Laracy," one of them quipped.

"We voted on Fluffett during the bus ride home," added Julie. "The name won hands down!"

I relaxed my authoritative stance and gave up the fight. I had learned to pick my battles. As if trying to soften the blow, Chris signaled for me to sit down and join their friends. For the next hour, Fluffett continued to entertain us to the point of ridiculousness. We Laracys had clearly been deprived of a furry pet for too long.

We were still in the throes of playtime when the doorbell rang. My mother and sister, Carol, had stopped by unannounced to meet our new pet. The house felt like New York City's Grand Central Station with all its visitors. Chris gently picked up the bunny and ran to open the front door, with Julie and me on his trail. He raised the bunny up like an offertory chalice and exclaimed, "Look how cute she is!" That would quickly become Chris's standard line when describing the bunny.

"She's a dwarf. A red satin named Fluffett. She'll only grow to weigh about two and a half pounds," I rattled off, sounding like I was reading a science report.

My mother looked at me the way a mother does sometimes, as if she knew before I ever would how much this bunny would bring our family together. "You were always rebellious," my mom said, glancing at the bunny. We both knew I had gotten my fire and spirit from her.

By the time darkness settled in, the neighborhood children had all gone home. Julie and Chris put Fluffett back in her cage, where she grazed on hay and let out all of her pent-up bodily waste. We tried to eat our dinner without being distracted. We would have to find a better location for her cage.

After finishing their dinner in record time, the children went to retrieve Fluffett, who darted toward the furthermost corner of her cage and ducked down for cover. But she had nowhere to hide.

"She might need a little more quiet time, kids," said my mom. The apple didn't fall far from the tree.

The poor kit would soon learn that there was no rest for the weary when it came to Chris. He reached into the cage from the top instead of the front latch, startling her. The bunny kicked litter up into the air and charged first to the right, then to the left, trying to dodge him.

"I can't catch her, Jules!" he yelled. The tiny bunny hopped over her bowl of food and bumped into the side of the cage trying to escape their grasp. She popcorned twice, ducked her head, and unknowingly lunged forward into Chris's waiting arms. She thrashed maniacally, her long furry hind paws scratching at his chest like snowshoes digging into the snow.

"Be careful of her back," I shrieked, remembering Loretta's warning. A rabbit's skeleton makes up only 7 percent of their body weight and is far more fragile than a dog's or a cat's. If a bunny swings its head backwards with too much force, it can fracture its own spine.

Hanging onto the bunny, Chris leapt up the stairs three steps at a time toward the playroom, ignoring me. Julie chased after him like someone had just stolen her favorite lip gloss.

"It's amazing how Flop survived her first week in the house with the five of you," said my mom, with a look that told me she had gone through this herself. "Pets are more resilient than you think, honey."

My mother's words always had a way of comforting me. I am not sure what I would have done without her and Carol in my life. They were strong, confident, and loving women, and we were completely devoted to each other. When I fell ill, their lives, too, were turned upside down. But heartache and sadness often draw families closer together. My mother became my private nurse, chief cook, and bottle washer; and Carol was her assistant. Some mornings, Mom would ring the doorbell at eight o'clock, carrying a casserole that she had already prepared for us to have for dinner that night. She would help out with breakfast and drive Chris to nursery school once Julie got on the bus, which conveniently stopped at the end of our driveway. My sweet little preschool boy and his adoring grandmother would walk out the front door hand in hand—Chris with his Batman backpack and Nana with her loving smile—as I pushed back my tears, unable to accept the fact that, at least for a while, I was physically broken. Instead I tried to focus on the miraculous bond that she and Chris were forming, which would remain indelible for the rest of their lives. On the nights that Ward had to work late, Carol would stop by on her way home from her job to help out with dinner and bath time for the kids and to offer her sisterly support and love, which I cherished. Carol and I had grown up sharing a bedroom, a wardrobe, our deepest confidences, and our hearts.

And so tonight was no different. My mother and sister were here to welcome the newest member of our family, witnesses to one of the most important and integral moments of our story.

"Can I help you clean the bunny's cage?" asked Carol, snapping me out of my daydreaming state. Mom also insisted on lending a hand. The McMansion was a mess and was already starting to smell. Shamelessly, I wasted no time taking up the offer. With the three of us working, the cleanup went quickly. We were piling fresh litter into the cage when hysterical sounds of laughter came roaring down from the family room. When we reached the top of the stairs, Chris was sitting on the floor with the bunny plopped on his lap. She was facing outward and resting on her haunches, as if she were sitting on a chair, while he clutched her torso.

"Mom, watch!" he exclaimed with a cunning "Dennis the Menace" look on his face. "She reminds me of a gumball machine."

The baby bunny was popping out little brown balls from the small opening between her back legs—perfectly synchronized, one per second. They fell into a neat pile between Chris's legs like raisinettes rolling off the assembly line into their box. The sideshow was so typical of Chris. He was mischievous and active, from the moment he was conceived, it seemed. He wreaked havoc on my body in utero, pounding my ribcage and most of my vital organs—and he was no different once he was born. Chris's milestones in his baby book read: "Scaled the baby gate," "climbed out of the highchair," "popped the inflatable swimming pool," and "third set of stitches," instead of things like, "Sat up," "rolled over," and "uttered his first word."

We lost count of the little brown balls after about forty. Carol glanced over at me as if to say, "Are you sure you know what you got yourself into?"

Fluffett's intelligence slowly began to show itself over and over again. She quickly fell into a daily routine. She would eat her baby bunny pellets made out of timothy hay around seven in the morning and six at night, while grazing on her hay around the clock. Unlike dogs, rabbits limit their intake of food and water, so Fluffett's supplies were plentiful. She had enough hay to feed a pony and enough water to survive a ten-year drought.

It seemed as if everything that went into Fluffett's body came out multiplied. By morning, her cage had enough brown pellets to supply an army of sharpshooters, and the smell of urine could burn the hairs inside of your nose. But thankfully, there were no cecotropes, which are grape-like clusters of soft, foul-smelling feces. Bunnies are supposed to ingest cecotropes to balance their intestinal flora—bunny probiotics. Sometimes I would spot Fluffett eating her probiotics, usually very early in the morning, dipping her head between her legs and plucking them from her butt.

My first attempt at litter-training Fluffett was partially successful. Once a rabbit picks their favorite place to urinate in, they can be taught to use a litter pan in that same spot. Fluffett had already peed in one corner of her cage.

It was a cold, damp, and dreary weekday. After reading the training instructions thoroughly, I filled the triangular litter pan from our bunny welcome package with pine shavings and placed it in the corner of the cage where she had been urinating. I left the bottom of the cage bare. The hard plastic bottom was supposed to be unappealing to our Baby Einstein. I piled some hay on top of the litter for Fluffett to munch on while she hopefully did her business, adding a few leaves of romaine lettuce on top as an extra incentive. Timothy hay, which should make up about 90 percent of a bunny's diet, is essential for proper digestion and helps grind down their teeth, which grow up to five inches a year. Fresh greens should only account for about 10 percent of a bunny's diet, as too much can cause diarrhea. I was already becoming a bunny expert.

By the time I finished prepping the cage, Fluffett was relaxing on the carpet by the back door. Her torso was flush against the floor and her legs were stretched out behind her like a pair of skis. Her hocks pointed toward the ceiling, and a perfectly shaped rear end formed at the juncture of her legs. She looked irresistible and perfectly content. I wondered if I should bother her or wait for another opportune moment to test her intelligence. But I was too excited. I wanted to surprise Julie and Chris when they got home from school.

"Let's try to litter train you, little girl." I said, curling up next to her. She nudged my cheek with the side of her head like a cat would and chinned me for the first time. Rabbits have scent glands on their chin. I was officially a marked woman.

Immediately, Fluffett sensed that something was different in her cage. She sniffed the plastic bottom curiously and bumped the litter pan with her head, trying to flip it over. She stood up on her hind legs and peered up through the top of the cage at me, looking befuddled.

"You're so smart, Fluffett," I exclaimed, the way I would if Julie or Chris had just handed me a great mid-term exam.

Fluffett flipped her head with a casualness that was endearing and hopped right into the litter pan. I giggled as she started tossing the lettuce up into the air like a baby seal knocking a ball. When the lettuce was torn to shreds, she sat down into what Julie called her Egyptian Sphinx position—I referred to it as Fluffett "plumping like a hen"—and nibbled on her hay.

I grabbed a pillow from the window seat in our kitchen and an *Arthritis Today* magazine, one of my reference guides on how to live with chronic pain, and sat on the floor next to her cage. Fluffett slowly devoured the lettuce first and then the entire pile of hay while she sat perched among the pine shavings. When she finally hopped out of the litter pan after about thirty minutes, there was a neat pile of poop pellets in the middle of the pine shavings. I jumped for joy, feeling a lightness I had not felt in a long time.

"Good job, Fluffett! I am so proud of you," I cried, bending down easily to kiss the top of her head, before catching myself. Usually, it wasn't easy for me to bend my body without feeling the pain.

Fluffett hopped along the plastic bottom as if playing hopscotch, but then she abruptly crouched down and peed there, outside of the litter pan. She slipped in the small puddle and looked around, confused. Hopping back into the pine shavings in the litter pan, she licked her now-yellow thumper paws (my affectionate name for her back paws), stretching each one up to her mouth like she was engaging in a yoga pose. She was cleaning herself like a cat would. Amazingly, her paws were white within minutes. Then she buried her head in her private parts and licked those until they, too, were pristine. I thought she was absolutely the cutest, smartest little bunny.

I sat back on the recliner with a feeling of great satisfaction and happiness, staring in awe at the newest member of our family, now cuddled in my arms. I rewarded her good behavior with a bunny snack, a corn stick, and fell back into my thoughts.

Strangely, I had barely noticed my pain all morning.

Chapter 5

I stared solemnly out my bedroom window past the melting patches of snow mixed among the winter grass, feeling guilty and heartbroken that our upcoming family vacation to Florida for winter break had to be postponed because of my health. As we were settling into our new lives with a rabbit, I was also battling a resurgence of extremely intense aches and pains. A flu virus had sent my connective tissue disease and fibromyalgia into a flare-up, and I was pummeled with crushing fatigue and unrelenting, intensified pain. The kind of pain that stops you in your tracks and puts your life on hold. Pain that can make you cry. It was frustrating and overwhelming living in constant fear that any virus, injury, or stressful event could turn manageable pain into something unmanageable.

The rheumatologist had started me on a large dose of steroids to curtail the inflammation in my system, and I struggled not to focus on my pain. I strongly believe that the mind plays an important role in how you perceive pain. In the past, I would have turned on soothing music or read a good book or soaked in the bathtub with lavender and Epsom salt—but now I played with our bunny. Holed up in the house, I set up elaborate mazes made out of sofa pillows, books, and baskets for Fluffett to race through. I made a bunny village out of cardboard boxes for her to rummage or hide in. I put empty toilet paper rolls and newspaper in her path and watched as her tiny teeth grabbed them and tried to toss them out of the way. I sprawled out on the floor and let her scamper all over me. I cuddled her against my chest while I answered emails or simply talked to her. I was smitten with our little bunny.

I had begun to recognize and understand some of Fluffett's habits, as well as her likes and dislikes. After she drank, she would shake her head or sneeze to get rid of any droplets of water that were on her whiskers. If I put hay in front of her and she wasn't hungry, she would burrow in the pile and toss the strands aside. When she sat back on her haunches with her head straight up and ears erect, it meant, "I'm here. Look at me." And we all did, nonstop. If she wanted to be petted, she would crouch down with her front paws forward and her chin and dewlap (the fur underneath a rabbit's chin) flush against the floor, waiting to be stroked. Our pet store bunny manual and the Internet both described the latter pose as the "submissive position," but Julie and I agreed that the name had to go.

When Fluffett was well rested and full of stored-up bunny energy, she would race around the sofas a dozen or more times with breakneck speed like a NASCAR driver until she tired herself out. She would literally fall over onto her side, making a thump. I ran over the first time she collapsed, fearing she'd had a heart attack. As prey animals on the bottom of the food chain, bunnies are high-strung and naturally fearful. Loud noises or sudden movements can frighten them, causing them to freeze or bolt. If they are terrified, they can literally drop dead from fear. But not our Fluffett, who loved the sound of the vacuum and thrived among the noise and commotion in our house.

Fluffett also made it clear when she wanted to relax and not be bothered. With no warning, she would sometimes sprawl out with her belly flush to the carpet, her head up, and her hind legs stretched behind her like a set of skis. The "leave me alone" position. As hard as that was, we respected her wishes.

The absolute cutest thing she did was to binky or popcorn. A bunny will start out hopping in one direction and then twist while in midair so it is facing another direction when it lands. If they do multiple binkies, you never know where they will end up. Their ability to binky and stop on a dime are convenient ways they use to escape predators. Fluffett could also wiggle into the smallest spaces as deftly as she had wiggled her way into our hearts. One day, I found her under Julie's desk nestled in one of her shoes.

Fluffett was smart, too. I attribute how Fluffett was able to figure out that Chris was the more sensitive and outwardly emotional child to the innate intelligence of rabbits. If she wanted to cuddle and hear how sweet or beautiful she was without any filter, Fluffett would scamper over to Chris, looking to be picked up. Conversely, when she was in a feisty mood, she would headbutt Julie's feet until Julie scooped her up under the armpits and nuzzled her face up against the bunny's twittering nose, saying to my horror, "You're cute. You're fat. You're really dumb, but I love you," in her sweetest candy-coated voice.

As far as Ward was concerned, his carefully orchestrated false indifference toward Fluffett disappeared the third or fourth day she was in the house. If she nuzzled on his shoe while he worked at his desk, he would reach down and give her an affectionate pet. Other times, he would put her on the desk and let her romp around with reckless abandon, disturbing his piles of papers.

Instinctively, Fluffett knew she had won my heart. I couldn't get enough of her as she twirled around the house, almost floating through the air like a ballerina. I turned a blind eye to her chewing and her mischief, enduring fierce criticism from my family. We kept a can of white trim paint nearby for all the moldings she nibbled and hung garbage bags on doorknobs for remnant pieces of household items she ruined. I picked up her stray brown pellets off the floor like they were dust balls and cleaned her cage with a smile, while I chastised Julie and Chris when their rooms were messy. I raced to the store when her yogurt drops ran low but often ran out of Ward's favorite ice cream. There were edible baskets and balls made out of hay scattered around the house, and she had a plastic bunny that wobbled from side to side. Whenever she learned a new task, such as coming when we called her or climbing up on our laps when we patted our thighs, we would put one yogurt drop inside the bunny, and the drop would pop out if she knocked into it. Bunny saltshakers and knickknacks were cropping up slowly around the house, driving Ward crazy. Ward hated clutter almost as much as he hated bickering.

It was a funny thing. This tiny rabbit had turned our house upside-down—or was it right-side-up? I couldn't help but wonder why I'd felt compelled to buy a rabbit that day in the middle of a blizzard, as if it meant something greater than anything I could imagine.

• • •

Like in previous years, Franklin Lakes would become a ghost town this time of the year when families would leave for the winter vacation—except for their pets. They were left behind. With most of our block away either at a warm destination or a ski resort, Chris capitalized upon all the opportunities to pet sit, and our Georgian colonial had been transformed into an exotic pet menagerie. He would make house calls on our street for the dogs or cats, and we would board the hamsters, lizards, and hermit crabs. Manson, our neighbor's vicious guinea pig, would be our main challenge. Chris was determined to tame him before the family returned from skiing. I hoped so—I had promised Chris, who was disappointed that we wouldn't be able to go on our annual vacation, that we would have a fun-filled staycation full of adventures. Luckily, I had Fluffett around to help.

Living in an affluent town had its advantages. Chris, with great forethought, took full advantage of the generosity of the Franklin Lakes families and upped the standard rate for pet sitting—a capitalist in the making. But with affluence also comes quirks. If your neighbor had a spaniel, they referred to their pooch as a Cavalier King Charles and got personally insulted if you called it anything else. And so it was that Fluffett became our "red satin of the lagomorph species" instead of just "a bunny."

A few days into the break, the house looked and smelled like a pet store. Cages were lined up in the kitchen and supplies were stacked in the hallway that led to the bathroom. It was a downright mess. Our moods had turned silly and relaxed from the additional rest and the absence of any scholastic or sports schedule. Feeding our never-ending appetites with homemade traditions, including our family-famous seven-layer magic bars, homemade Mickey Mouse waffles, cinnamon buns, and grilled cheeses made with three different cheeses, tomato, and avocado, made everyone more jovial. Food played a crucial role in the Laracy family. Eating was not just a basic need for our household of four; it was an experience in itself. We often called ourselves the *Food Family*, and we demonstrated our culinary obsession with elaborate, themed parties I often threw, complete with customized homemade goods.

Keeping track of the feeding schedule for the animals was no small task, but it was fun. Chris made sure that we stayed on track and that no one was overfed. Except us Laracys.

"I handle all the snacks while the animals are under my care," Chris said with a seriousness that told us not to question his authority. "Rules are rules." He was determined for his new endeavor to be successful and for word to get out that he was a competent pet sitter. Being the ultimate rule-breaker himself, Chris's comment puzzled but charmed me.

Because our week had become all about the animals, I decided to make a second attempt at litter training Fluffett with the help of the children, since our first run had only been partially successful. Julie and Chris ran to find the video camera, giving Fluffett a pep talk and sounding like cheerleaders for the middle school basketball team, while I prepared her cage. Our moods couldn't be dampened even when we realized the video camera wasn't working. We just focused on the task on hand.

Fluffett skipped the curious, incessant sniffing around her cage that she had done the first time. She hopped into the litter pan and plumped in it, sitting like a sphinx again. We watched patiently while she munched on her hay furiously, the hay disappearing quickly as if it were being sucked into a wood chipper instead of a one-pound rabbit. With a lone strand left, Fluffett leaned forward on her front paws like she was about to do a handstand. Then, she very deliberately lifted her hind end up and peed.

Our applause rivaled anything I had heard at the US Open. I looked over at Chris and mouthed silently, "Baby Einstein." Julie and Chris held hands and gazed at their baby bunny with obvious pride, their faces glowing.

Fluffett knew she had done something good. She pranced around her cage with her head high, turning it from side to side like she was modeling an Easter bonnet. Then she binkied in several directions and spun so high that she crashed into the top of her cage. Instantly, she transformed from "happy" bunny to "hostile" bunny, like I had been accused of doing at times. Clawing at the rungs of the cage, she bared her teeth for the first time. Our domestic bunny had gone postal. Chris swept her up and tried to calm her down by stroking the ultra soft spot behind her ears. She thumped her hind legs on his chest, making a loud noise. Rabbits thump when they are frightened, angry, or in pain; or if they want to demand your attention. We would learn much later that a non-dwarf, fully grown rabbit could have broken Chris's ribs by thumping.

Chris tightened his grasp just enough to keep Fluffett from falling and whispered into her sandy-colored ears while he softly kissed the side of her face. "Good job, Fluffett. You're the best bunny in the world."

Fluffett dropped her head and nuzzled it between the buttons on his shirt. Her body relaxed instantly. Julie and I joined in Fluffett's praise, reciting enough positive adjectives to write a bunny thesaurus. Fluffett began pawing at Chris's buttons playfully. She flipped her tiny body in three or four different directions before burrowing in his lap like she was digging for gold. She rolled over on her back, her hind legs and front paws pointing upward, like a big old—dare I say the word—*dog*.

Then Chris committed the cardinal sin: he started rubbing the gauzy fur on her belly. Rabbits hate to have their bellies or chins rubbed, and I fully expected Fluffett to bolt. Instead, before my own eyes, she raised her four legs up and spread them outward, prostrate, like any attention-seeking dog, and fell into a trance. We watched in total disbelief. Chris had gotten the dog he always wanted; it had just come disguised as a rabbit.

For the next few weeks, Fluffett's litter habits were unpredictable. She had stopped peeing on hard surfaces, but soft surfaces were still a crapshoot. She slipped up one night while she was lying on my chest. I had on my softest Old Navy hooded fleece sweatshirt. Ward and I were watching *The Sopranos*.

"What can I say? The show is too violent!" I joked when I felt the warm liquid seep through the fleece.

Chapter 6

Spring was soon upon us. Purple and yellow crocuses poked up from the ground and small patches of green grass pushed their way through the old, matted-down winter grass. The sun had resumed its seasonal position in the sky, bringing with it more daylight and warmth, which never failed to improve my outlook on life. Mounds of snow had finally melted, giving us hope that spring would actually arrive on schedule.

In March, I dedicated my time and energy to planning Julie's twelfth birthday party. The theme was *American Idol*, our family's guilty pleasure and the show we loved to watch together, just as the Buchalskis would gather to watch *The Monkees* and *The Partridge Family* when I was a child. Birthdays were a big event in our house, a tradition I inherited from my childhood home. Having a near-Christmas birthday on December 19 didn't make it any less special for me. Mom and Dad always made sure I had a themed party, plenty of presents, and my favorite meal—simple breaded chicken cutlets, homemade French fries, and strawberry short-cake. To carry on the tradition that gave me so much joy, each year I would put my creative talents to the test, organizing themed parties such as Care Bears, My Little Ponies, Power Rangers, Pokémon, and Batman. And of course, since we were the Food Family, birthday parties were a chance for me to show off my culinary skills.

Despite this year's *American Idol* theme, Julie had a primary focus: Fluffett, who ended up taking center stage. I brushed Fluffett's fur, which had thickened significantly, smoothed her ears, and tied a pink, sparkly sequined bow around her neck. Fluffett was my chance to indulge in my girlish nature. I felt like I was primping one of Julie's old American Girl Dolls!

I changed my clothes, thinking that life with a bunny on boar
was proving to be very different than any of us had imagined. Fluffet
unknowingly, was offering us some unique bunny wisdom about how
make the best of things and showing us why life is great with a bun*
around.

To my delight, Fluffett was admired by all the guests. Our house was filled with loud, incessant giggling—over my artfully crafted cake that was supposed to resemble a microphone but that turned out to look more like a part of the male anatomy I cannot mention!—to loud and theatrical amateur karaoke and fun-filled dancing. Simon Cowell would certainly have made some harsh comments. Meanwhile, Fluffett bounced around the family room like she was on a trampoline, sniffing purses or tossing shoes with her teeth, all while tripping on wires and tripping the girls.

After an ill-fated and temporary jaunt in our outdoor jacuzzi—the girls' splashes had caused water to overflow, cutting the electricity—and a last hurrah of "swimsuit karaoke," the party drew to a close. It was finally time to rest. My body ached from head to toe from all the party planning and preparations, but it was worth it for Julie. I retreated to the bedroom and let myself fall backward onto the bed, forcing a just-as-exhausted Fluffett to hang out with me on our luscious down comforter.

I kissed her fluffy tail. I did noogies on the top of her head and made loud raspberries on the side of her face. I whispered, "I love you, my little girl. Your round little rump, your wiggling nose, and your furry thumper paws." Fluffett tried to escape my affections, so I let her wriggle free. She burrowed into the blue-and-white floral comforter, as she would have in the wild. She tried to flip the throw pillows with her head, but they ended up on top of her. "Peek a boo!" I exclaimed, lifting them off. I scooped her up and tucked her in between my knees, and she laid on her back while I rubbed her belly. Then she wriggled away to burrow again. Was she trying to burrow her way to freedom or safety? I let her use up some of her baby energy and watched as deep crevices began to form all over the comforter. When I grabbed her from behind playfully, she scurried onto my chest and relaxed her thumper paws. Either she'd realized her attempts to flee were futile or she was tiring out. She nibbled the sequins on my blouse, pulling one or two off. It was just like having a baby again. The warmth and softness of her body was the perfect remedy for my sore muscles. I could feel the stress almost evaporating from my body as I became oblivious to my surroundings.

"Am I interrupting something?"

I looked up, embarrassed. Ward was standing in the doorway. I wasn't sure how long he had been there.

"Fluffett and I were just relaxing."

He raised his eyebrows, skeptically.

"I'm not gonna lie. I was telling Fluffett how special she was."

"I heard it all, Nance. *I* should be that lucky," he replied, with all the bite of a stand-up comedian.

•   •   •

Before we knew it, it was Easter. The tips of the cherry trees looked like they had been dipped in icing, their pink and white buds waiting to burst open. The canopy of green from the oak trees that would soon blanket our yard was beginning to form.

It was a beautiful, sundrenched April day. The house was still quiet. Fluffett and I were sitting together on the wingback chair next to the fireplace in the living room. Through the window, fair weather clouds were floating across the bright blue sky. The sound of birds chirping outside filled the room.

I savored the snugness of her furry body. Her back paws and belly leaned close against my breastbone while her face and front paws nestled in my neck. I talked to her about many things. My Easter memories as a child. My health challenges. Some of our crazier Laracy moments. And Flop. A feeling of contentment had wrapped itself around me and Fluffett. My heart melted with happiness as she purred for the first time—the subtle vibration against my skin felt delicious. From everything I had read, purring is a rare expression of a rabbit's deep love. It is a sign of utter bliss, which described the way I, too, felt at that moment.

I thought about my Easters as a child. While I loved rummaging through my Easter basket, I was almost as excited to see the dress and matching coat and hat my mother had made for my sister and me, using the beautiful wool and cotton fabrics her sister sent her every year for Christmas. I can still remember the look of joy on my mother's face when that large brown box arrived every year in mid-December. Her eyes would light up, dreaming of the clothes she would be able to make for us girls and herself. Mom was a beautiful seamstress, and she loved to sew. "I am happy when I am sewing," she would say, leaning over her Singer machine. She did most of sewing at night when we were in bed. "Don't stay up too late, Anne," my dad would say. But we knew she did.

That Easter in the Laracy home, Julie and Chris came rushing downstairs to three Easter baskets on our kitchen counter. They were brimming over with candy and other sundries.

"There's a basket for Fluffett!" I could hear the surprise and happiness in their voices.

"Happy Easter!" they shrieked, hopping across the living room like two jack rabbits. Chris whisked Fluffett up without any warning, kissed my cheek, and carried her into the kitchen to see her bright-pink and lime-green woven basket full of bunny treats. The table was already set for breakfast—four pastel-colored placemats in yellow, green, lavender, and pink, along with matching plates. On one end of the table, I had placed porcelain rabbit salt and pepper shakers; to the left of the plates were matching porcelain bunny napkin rings stuffed with striped pastel cloth napkins my mother had made for me when we were first married. I always took special care to create a welcoming home for my family. It gave me great pleasure.

Ward rounded the corner in time to see Chris show Fluffett her very first Easter basket. She bypassed the giant economy-sized box of yogurt drops, egg-shaped wicker treats, and other items I had given great time and thought to purchasing, and instead lunged toward the chocolate in the kid's baskets with an infectious enthusiasm that only a bunny can muster on Easter.

"Grab her!" I screamed. Julie caught Fluffett in midair just as she was about to topple off the counter.

"If she falls, she can break her back," I blurted out, a sense of panic rushing over me. "And she can't have the chocolate. Caffeine can give her a heart attack." Just as it is for dogs, chocolate is deadly for rabbits.

"Chill, Mom, I caught her," said Julie, shrugging. "And do you really think we would give up our chocolate without a fight?" She grinned. "Happy Easter."

"Let's take some pictures with Fluffett," said Chris, unable to control his excitement.

Did I hear him right? I thought to myself. Julie and Chris always hated having their pictures taken. But this was their first Easter with a real rabbit. Even their baskets of candy took a back seat.

Our Easter photoshoot was like something right out of Hollywood. We took dozens of creative (and not-so-creative) photos of our new rabbit. Fluffett plumped in her basket. Fluffett on the piano bench beside some sheet music. Fluffett cuddled up on the sofa with a stuffed rabbit. Fluffett perched behind the fireplace screen. Julie and Chris were in a few of the pictures, but make no mistake, Fluffett was the main star. She was Diana Ross, and the kids were happy to be the background singers.

Finally, I asked if I could be in one of the photos.

Like a seasoned mother, I cradled Fluffett against my soft pink blouse, and a lone tear of joy trailed down my cheek. Life had changed so much for us in such a short time. I truly believed that our enchanting bunny was a gift from God—and she would be for more reasons that I would soon come to realize. A gift we had learned to nurture and dote on. A gift who brought so much joy and relief to our lives. And a gift whose list of potential babysitters, while we planned to go away for our spring break vacation, would become longer than the Food Family's weekly grocery list.

• • •

During previous vacations, we had boarded Sunny, our Australian bearded dragon, at the pet store Scuffy's due to her unusual diet of live worms and crickets, which deterred friends and family from pet sitting. But boarding Fluffett was never an option. She needed much more socialization and exercise than Sunny, who preferred to spend the bulk of her time basking contentedly on a log or under her sunlamp. Fluffett commanded our full attention, unless she was napping. I suppose I had taught her to be that way.

My mother and sister, who lived together, would have been the perfect choice to pet sit Fluffett, except for the fact that they had a cat. Every spring, their friendly, domestic feline turned into a wild animal on the prowl for poor defenseless kits huddled in their nests. Each season, Tigergirl would carry one or two baby bunnies home in her jaws and drop them on the porch with a look of satisfaction. Just the thought of it made me shudder.

As the days passed, the vetting process became intense. The discussions turned hostile. We all had a different opinion on who fit the bill. Finally, I used my veto power to pick the one family in town who met the rigorous standards I had set. Keith and Cindy Funsch, our clean and nurturing churchgoing neighbors, had two lovely, calm children and no predatory pets. The other contender, my neighbor Karen, was a past bunny owner who vied for the assignment, claiming to have far better credentials. However, vivid tales of her outdoor rabbit, Jaws, and Manson the notorious guinea pig hindered her chances. Less-than-cordial phone calls had been exchanged between Karen and the Funsch family, and by the time we dropped Fluffett off at the Funsches', the neighbors were barely speaking.

"We're honored to have her," said Cindy, as the kids and I paraded into her kitchen.

"Where would you like the cage?" Chris asked politely, slipping and crashing into the kitchen counter—making me cringe as I quickly apologized. Julie dragged in a duffle bag on wheels that was full of Fluffett's supplies. I carried the princess.

"You're coming back, right?" Cindy asked, eyeing the humongous duffle bag.

"It's just a few things." I smiled.

Cindy and I moved to the family room to discuss the more elaborate details of Fluffett's care. As I took the list of elaborate instructions and phone numbers where we could be reached out of my pocket, I chuckled at my own madness and ridiculous rules.

"Now," I said, turning and looking into her eyes to make sure I had her full attention, "a rabbit needs different care than a dog or cat."

Instructions for Fluffett's Care

1. Never leave Fluffett alone or unattended when she is out of her cage. She'll chew almost anything, valuable or not. Keep her away from wires and stairs. They're both off limits. Please don't undermine me!
2. Never discipline Fluffett.
3. Please don't pick Fluffett up by the scruff of her neck. She is not a wild rabbit. Support her hind legs. Be careful that she doesn't use your sofa as a trampoline to bounce off—and fall and break her back. Rabbits are fragile creatures. Feel free to snuggle with her, but in moderation. Remember, I'm her mother.
4. Empty the litter pan daily and clean with the Johnson's Baby Soap, which is also in the duffle bag. Keep the pink blanket on the top of the cage at night because she loves her blankie. Don't substitute one of yours as she will chew it to shreds through the rungs of the cage.
5. Fill her food bowl halfway daily with timothy hay pellets and pile a ginormous amount of hay on top of her litter. She's not a pony, but she grazes like one.
6. She can have the carrot tops in the small cooler as a treat, but not the carrots. I repeat, the tops only, not the whole carrot. Carrots have too much sugar and will give her diarrhea. I never did trust Bugs Bunny.
7. Feel free to give Fluffett some of her new chew toys, which are buried somewhere among her other supplies. The pink raspberry-flavored yogurt drops need to be rationed. Only one a day. They're candy, cleverly named, and packaged to appear healthy.
8. Fill the water bottle with fresh, cold water each day. She snubs her nose if the water is room temperature. Bottled water is fine!
9. Use the sound machine when you go to bed. Rabbits are crepuscular animals. Yes, that's a big, new word, right? That

means they are very active between dusk and dawn. She won't be sleeping while you are—trust me.

Thanks so much and have fun!

I looked up with a silly grin. "That should do it. Any questions?"

"Just make sure that your cell phone is charged," Cindy laughed.

We walked back to the kitchen where Julie, Chris, and the Funsch children were sitting on the floor watching Fluffett acclimate to her surroundings. Toys were already scattered around the kitchen, and Fluffett was popcorning around the bar stools that surrounded the granite island.

"It's time to leave," I said glumly. Almost instantly, Julie and Chris had the same pained look on their faces. We could barely tear ourselves away. Fluffett would no doubt spend her first day at the Funsches' licking off the saliva from all our kisses. The lengthy, tearful goodbye reminded me of the day my baby brother, Tom, and his new wife, Audrey, moved to Colorado, leaving the rest of us siblings behind. You would have thought that they were going into exile and that we would never see them again. For better or for worse, my extended family and I were inseparable. We lived close geographically, and our hearts were intertwined. Before Tom moved out west, we siblings had all lived within ten miles of each other. We spent so much of our time together. We would tailgate at West Point Military Academy and go pumpkin or apple picking in the fall. During the winter, we would cut down our Christmas trees together and have "Breakfast with Santa" at one of the children's schools or go on a train ride through western New Jersey. In the spring, we picnicked at Van Saun Park and hiked to the lake at the top of Ramapo Ridge. We attended each other's children's sporting events or dance recitals whenever possible and organized painting parties when someone's house needed sprucing up. Our bond was indelible, for which we credited our wonderful parents. I routinely thanked my mother for raising five loving and caring children, and I spoke to my father gratefully each day in prayer. I would play my father's favorite song, "Moon River" by Henry Mancini, on my iPod or pop in the CD I kept in my car whenever I wanted to feel close to him.

So when the kids and I reluctantly finished our goodbyes and left the Funsches', I played "Moon River" as we drove away. The lyrics never failed to make me happy.

After dropping Sunny off at Scuffy's, I suggested getting ice cream at Baskin Robbins. I had an ulterior motive—Baskin Robbins shared a space with Dunkin' Donuts, and I was dying for a hot cup of coffee and also needed to stock up on supplies. I had used up the last grinds, and the thought of not having my morning coffee before we left for the airport the next day was dreadful. A steaming hot cup of half-caffeinated coffee was a comfort drink for me, in particular on the mornings when I woke up immersed in the classic "fibro fog," a symptom of fibromyalgia that can be described as seeing the world through the milky cover of cataracts. The heat from the mug helped unstiffen my sore hands, and the caffeine would begin to peel away the white veil that was seemingly draped over my eyes. Within fifteen minutes, I would be able to see and process the world with more clarity. Over the last six years, I rolled over every morning yearning for my java. And now, I had Fluffett, too! Already, I missed her. I couldn't wait to feel her furry paws scurrying over my feet and her twittering nose tickling my toes again.

On the day of our departure to Florida, the pitter-patter of rain on the windows woke me prematurely. I walked quietly downstairs, hoping to organize some last-minute things to ensure a timely, peaceful exit. Getting ready for a big vacation in the Laracy household was intense. There was often chaos and missteps. Ward would jump in at the ninth hour after working an iron day and squeeze his worldly belongings into a small suitcase without breaking a sweat. But packing for the remaining three of us, arranging care for the animals, and micromanaging every detail of the trip was my job. Simple tasks like taking clothes out of drawers or off hangers to cram into a suitcase caused my body to throb. I would have to pace myself and take four Advils. By the time we got to our destination, I was usually ready for more than one welcome drink.

The kitchen felt empty that morning without Fluffett and her cage. A long row of suitcases was arranged along the wall—nine bags of all sizes. I had tried to keep my packing light—five pairs of sandals to go with ten outfits—but Julie didn't try. She had her own opinion now on how she dressed. "Two bathing suits, some shorts, and a couple of T-shirts—that's all you need," an exact quote from her father, was not what she had in mind when she packed her suitcase to a point where the zipper almost split open.

We left home on schedule. The traffic was light on the roads, despite the slow, steady rain. Within six hours we were lying on a beach, soaking up the Florida sun. I had already called home twice to check on Fluffett—once when I dodged into the bathroom, feigning an oncoming irritable bowel attack while everyone changed into their bathing suits, and again when I offered to get everyone's beach towels at the towel hut on the other side of the pool. Fluffett was fine.

Our destination, Marco Island, was a lovely, tropical suburb on the South Gulf coast. Our hotel was located on the beach, overlooking a long jetty that harbored crabs and other crustaceans. The ocean had tiny waves—more like ripples—which disappointed Ward and the kids. Seagulls flew overhead, dotting the blue skies. Colorful umbrellas and sand toys filled the sprawling beaches, and families were everywhere. The swim-up bar was standing room only and the line for the pool floats seemed to be an over-thirty crowd. There was a nature center brilliantly and strategically placed between the beach and the pool, where children could handle crawly creatures or watch nature videos. Next to the nature center was the "arts and craps" center, Julie's nickname for the colorful, whimsical room where children could stop in to show off their creative talents.

After three days of relaxation, sunshine, and 84° weather, my maintenance dose of the steroid prednisone for joint and muscle pain, which defined my existence, had decreased significantly, and I was feeling more energetic. Less stress and warm weather can temporarily lessen the pain of fibromyalgia, though not necessarily my connective tissue pain, which depends on how my immune system is working at a certain time and how much inflammation is going on inside my body. Having a connective tissue disease is often difficult to explain to most people as it is a combination of lupus and rheumatoid arthritis—essentially, your body has not yet differentiated which full-blown disease you have. At times, I found myself telling others that I had lupus, what most people are painfully familiar with.

I strolled the beaches with Julie and Chris collecting seashells, got caught up on Hollywood gossip reading *People* magazine, and drained the battery of my iPod listening to my music: theme songs from Rodgers and Hammerstein's *Cinderella*, Andrew Lloyd Weber's *The Phantom of the Opera*, and various tunes by Jimmy Buffett, Bob Marley, the Monkees, and the Partridge Family. And, of course, "Moon River," sung by Andy Williams. I had also racked up over forty minutes on my cell phone, checking on Fluffett. She was still doing fine.

Everyone was having a great time, except for Ward. His cell phone had not stopped ringing with business issues long enough for him to take a leisurely swim or read more than one chapter of his book. I could see his frustration mounting.

He broke the news to us over lunch.

"I have to leave, Nance. You and the kids can stay. There's no sense ruining the trip for all of us."

I looked at him, heartbroken. Our winter trip had been canceled due to my health, and now this!

"But Dad, you can't leave!!" Chris erupted, springing out of his chair.

"I'm so sorry, kids. It is out of my control." Ward gathered us into a family huddle. As a corporate transactional attorney, Ward was often at the mercy of whatever merger or acquisition he was working on. But being the great sport and wonderful provider for his family that he was, he took it in his stride.

"I'll see you at home in a few days. I can make arrangements to help your mom with the luggage on the trip back," Ward said. He knew how painful it might be for me to lug all the suitcases myself.

"I can handle it," I replied softly. Hiding my weaknesses from the children was my modus operandi. This time was no different; I *would* manage.

Julie and Chris's negotiations with their father continued well into the evening, but they were unsuccessful. He left on a seven o'clock flight the following morning.

"Oh well, Dad's gone," said Chris when he stumbled out of bed a few hours later, not content to dwell on the change of plans. "Party time."

Dashing into the bedroom, he grabbed the pillow out from under Julie's head and tossed it across the room. I rounded the corner in time to get a mouthful of feathers. Engaging my reflexes, I quickly threw the pillow straight back at him. He dodged my throw, but Julie, a chip off of the old block, jumped out of bed and wrestled him to the ground with one impressive sweep. I had taught her my technique. Growing up with three brothers, I had learned early on that brute strength could only be matched with skill, agility, and speed.

While Julie and Chris enjoyed the vacation time spent with their dad, they knew I had a propensity for being silly and would always be up for a bit of senseless, exhilarating fun. When we were done with our impromptu pillow fight, we pushed the tousled hair out of our eyes and straightened our disheveled clothes. With Julie and me decked out in our bug-eyed sunglasses and wide-brimmed hats, the three of us walked out of the room and down the hallways, incognito, like celebrities, dodging the cleaning staff.

At the pool, I called to check on Fluffett while Julie and Chris tried to drown each other over a shortage of pool floats. Cindy picked up the phone on the fourth ring.

"How's Fluffett doing, Cindy?"

"Who's this?"

"It's Nancy."

"I know who it is. It was you the last time and the time before. Fluffett's fine, Nance. I was just following her up the stairs when the phone rang."

I wanted to scream, "I said *no* stairs!" Instead, I said, "Are you keeping an eye on her?"

"Of course," she said enthusiastically. "Fluffett lets herself in and out of her cage, and she knows her way around downstairs. She also learned how to go up the stairs on the first try."

In and out of her cage? Up the stairs? I was intrigued. We had never left the door of Fluffett's cage open, mainly for safety reasons. It had never dawned on me that we might eventually allow her unsupervised freedom. I had chosen the Funsches for their conservative parenting techniques, but they were obviously closet liberals!

"Thanks for taking such good care of her," I said, hanging up the phone.

As I wandered back to the pool, I was tickled pink by the idea of letting Fluffett roam more freely throughout the house. I could feel excitement bundling up inside of me. Suddenly, the idea of going back to the damp, cool spring weather, which greatly exacerbates my pain, didn't seem so bad. I had a bunny adventure waiting for me!

A spontaneous, last-minute daytrip to the Florida Everglades ended up being a highlight of our trip, second only to the pillow fight. Our maniacal airboat guide with his "Captain Crazy" hat and boat slithered through the murky water of the Everglades. Alligators big and small lurked beneath the dark swamp water, popping up a little too close to the boat for Julie and me.

"Keep your hands in the boat if you want to go home with two," said Captain Crazy as Chris leaned over the boat, pointing to a group of gators. "He's a typical boy, Mom," the captain said for my benefit. "Just try to relax."

We, or rather Chris, topped off the trip with a photo opportunity, where he posed clutching a baby gator as if he were Steve Irwin. The following morning, we boarded our seven o'clock flight home. Our flight was packed with snowbirds—senior citizens who lived up north in the spring and summer and who flew south for warmer weathers during the winter. Chris, who had spent many afternoons as a toddler frequenting senior citizen meetings with my mother when I was sick, turned into a one-man comedy show, roaming the aisles and cracking jokes. Julie was on his heels, an ambassador of goodwill, doling out compliments like, "I just love your hair" or "Lavender is definitely your color." The snowbirds were definitely enchanted with Julie and Chris; I wondered what they'd have thought of Fluffett!

It was pouring rain and thirty-nine miserable degrees when our plane landed in Newark, the armpit of otherwise beautiful New Jersey. Midway through the long walk to the baggage "clam," as Julie liked to call it, I was already limping in pain. The change happened that fast. I was destined to retire to a warm, dry climate.

We charged the Funsches' front door like trick or treaters fighting over a bucket of candy. When we stepped inside, Fluffett poked her head around the kitchen corner, her big ears standing tall. Then she popcorned almost in a straight line across the entrance foyer toward the stairway leading to the second floor. She hopped onto the first step, sat upright on her haunches, and stared at us. I wondered why she didn't come rushing over and worried she had forgotten who we were; perhaps she was mad we had left her.

Julie and Chris scooped Fluffett up and took turns holding her, nearly as excited as the night we first bought her. When it was my turn, I reveled in the softness of her fur. Her fluttering whiskers felt like a gentle Florida breeze on my cheek. I had missed our kit so much.

"What have you been up to, silly girl?" I asked. "Mischief, I think?" I looked at Cindy.

"Fluffett loves having her freedom," said Cindy, hanging her head, as if admitting that she had overlooked some of the rules. My instruction "Don't Undermine Me!" must have not been written in bold letters.

At last, we could go home with our baby bunny.

Chapter 7

"Little Bunny foo foo sitting in the poo poo! Little Bunny foo foo sitting in the poo poo!"

I found myself routinely singing a silly tune to Fluffett whenever she plumped in her litter pan. As I sang, I thought, *My god, what's happening to me?* I had completely fallen in love with our charming, mischievous little rabbit. The supposedly shy creature who now headbutted my feet or thumped her hind legs demanding to be picked up; the bunny who whacked the phone if I tried to speak to someone while we were cuddling; the feisty, playful rabbit who would untie my sneakers with her front teeth or belly crawl across the sofa and nibble at my socks or the remote control.

I had volunteered to teach supplemental Spanish at Chris's grammar school, but my lesson plans had taken a back burner because of our furry friend's distractions. I resorted to ad-libbing and retrieving vocabulary and grammar from my long-term memory, which was, fortunately, sharp as a tack. As a child, the nuns at my Catholic grammar school told my parents they thought I had close to a photographic memory. And that I talked too much. Ward and the kids doubted the first statement, but nuns don't lie. When we heard the same phrase "photographic memory" at Julie's fifth grade teacher conference, the family's skepticism about my memory faltered.

Having a great memory made things easier in many ways. When I was in grade school, times tables, division, spelling, and most facts found their way into my long-term memory with great ease. During high school I was able to work two jobs at a time and still maintain good grades, while many of my friends struggled to study and hold down one job. Prior to motherhood, my twelve-year career in executive recruiting was the perfect vocation for a girl with a chatty personality and a good memory. I could spend an hour interviewing a prospective job applicant, make a few mental notes, and four years later be able to retrieve their information from my brain instead of the filing cabinet. I could remember their personality, education, and work history; what suit, skirt, or hairstyle they wore; and whether or not they had on lipstick or aftershave. I knew who ran what departments within specific corporations and what their salary structure and benefits were without searching through a single job requisition. I worked in a third of the time of the average recruiter, earning top dollar for myself. I ignored the occasional sexist comment dealt to me, such as, "Wear that black skirt with the side slit when you meet the president of ADP" or "Don't forget to wear your lipstick," and I reaped the benefits of being one of the first successful women in the tri-state area in that particular male-dominated business. I never had to pay for a business lunch or dinner and was showered with gifts around the holidays and my birthday.

Now, as I spent my afternoons teaching rote memorization to young school children, I knew it would never be as lucrative as my work in Human Resources. But the happiness and fulfillment I felt with being involved in my children's schools meant so much to me. I loved being a stay-at-home mom.

By the end of the school year, my young prodigies had a strong command of Spanish. They could recite their names and ages, as well as what their favorite foods were. They could tell me whether they were "*contento o triste*" (happy or sad), where they lived, and whether or not they liked watching television or reading books. They also knew a few random words like *conejo*—bunny!

On the home front, Fluffett was starting to understand the words we spoke and getting better with each passing day. When I called out, "Fluffett, do you want to go for a ride in the car?" she would scurry out from wherever she was and binky in a small circle around my feet—almost bouncing. Once we were in the car, depending on the time of day, she would roll over and relax on the front seat—the motion of the car putting her almost into a trance—or stretch her body up against the door to look out the window, which she could still barely reach. I cradled her in my left arm while I ran mundane errands like going to the post office or the dry cleaner's. We intrigued proprietors wherever we went, and I wasn't shy about striking up a conversation about my lagomorph!

Fluffett and I had also discovered a game we loved to play—the Bunny Game. It took place in the living room, which was, ironically, off limits to the kids to play in. Rabbits have very good memories and quickly form routines and patterns of behavior. Fluffett would sprawl out on her belly in the archway leading into the room and wait for me to clap my hands.

"Fluffett, do you want to play the Bunny Game?"

She would set out in frenzy, hopping around the legs of the piano and the coffee tables. She'd squeeze under the sofa and fly out from the other side, running behind the fireplace screen to catch her breath. I would creep up slowly and clap again. "Where's the bunny?" She'd charge out with renewed zest and popcorn across the room out of sheer happiness. I am not sure who enjoyed the game more, she or I.

By midsummer, Fluffett was completely litter trained. She had given up chewing on the things she shouldn't after Chris scolded her forcibly for shredding his Nintendo wires. The "shock and awe" seemed to have worked; I could have taken parenting lessons from Chris. Without needing our supervision, Fluffett now had free rein over an entire house. Once she figured out that our Georgian colonial was just a giant habitat for her to play in, more aspects of her quirky, endearing personality emerged. She hopped her way through various rooms, settling in preferred spots at different times of the day. She enjoyed stretching out under the dining room chairs in the late morning or on the lower shelves of the plant stands in the sunroom during the afternoon.

Bunnies are least active during the day, and Fluffett loved to nap, especially in the sunroom. Ceramic bunnies lined the edge of the two moss-green wooden steps that led down into the room. A stuffed sandy-brown bunny that wore different themed sweaters for Easter, Christmas, and July Fourth—a Mother's Day gift from my sister—sat on the green chenille sofa. Three papier-mâché bunnies, a mother and two babies—Ward's gift to me after attending a charity event at the Metropolitan Museum of Art—stood on top of the armoire. And Fluffett was most comfortable buried among the vast array of new "indestructible" silk plants and flowers (initially, she had torn our old fake plants to shreds as quickly as I'd kill the real ones). Fluffett soaked up the sun's rays as they poured through the tall windows. Her ginger-colored fur shimmered exquisitely and her dark eyes sparkled like black diamonds. As the shadow of the sun edged its way across the carpet and settled on the wooden floor, she would sniff out cozier pastures. And once she was well rested, she was ready for some serious playtime.

For the next few hours, she would be underfoot, seeking attention from us or playing by herself. When we were all gathered upstairs in the family room, she'd roll around in her wicker tunnel filled with hay, nearly flipping upside down, or she'd knock her toys in our path, inviting us to play with her. Then, as Julie and Chris's bedtime approached, like clockwork, Fluffett would exit the family room, hopping slowly down the stairs one step at a time, hoping we wouldn't see her sneak out.

Fluffett had already figured out that Ward's and my bedtime was not much later than the children's, which meant she would soon be put in her cage. Though I now trusted Fluffett to roam free during the day, I still wasn't completely comfortable with letting her run free at night. Fluffett hated to be locked up. Some bunnies find comfort in their cozy warren, but not our rabbit. When Fluffett began her nightly descent down the stairs, one of us would follow her. She would dart across the hard kitchen floor and hide under the dining room table, hoping to put off being put in her cage. I found her habits and perception of time intriguing.

Over time, we worked out a playful routine to catch her. Initially, we tried to outrun her. We would surround the table, each of us at our different posts, while Fluffett weaved through the legs of the table and chairs with the speed and agility of a black diamond skier. We had to be careful how we grabbed her, assuming we were able to, due to her frail musculoskeletal structure, but time and time again she escaped our grasp. We tried waving pieces of apple and yogurt drops in front of her, but she quickly learned not to take the bait. Fluffett was cunning, and before she ran out of steam, she would change strategies, charging forward as if about to come out from one side of the table and stopping short before we could grab her, causing her back end to nearly flip over her head, which was absolutely adorable. She looked like a tuft of ginger-colored cotton blown up into the air. She would then popcorn back the way she had come, clearly trying to fool us. Most times, she did.

We finally realized that we needed to tire her out, which took time. Luckily, Julie and Chris had plenty of it—they hated bedtime, just like our rabbit. And despite the fact that, by the end of the day, my joint and muscle pain would have increased significantly from performing simple daily tasks like emptying the dishwasher, reaching for the pocketbook, or setting the dinner table, I was always more than happy to get down on the rug. It was all part of the game.

We would sit at our posts and wait. And wait. Eventually, Fluffett would tire herself out. Once she started to binky in slow motion, I knew she was winding down. Julie and Chris would say goodnight, and I would lie there, perfectly still, sometimes for close to ten minutes, waiting patiently for the end of the game. The lawyer in our house would say, "Nance, close the deal."

Inching her furry little front paws out, Fluffett would creep out on her belly, butt up, like a tiger ready to pounce. Stealthily, she would slowly and thoroughly sniff my entire torso, from toe to head. When her whiskers tickled my nose, I would snatch her up.

"Gotcha, silly girl!"

It worked every time. By that point, I think she wanted to be caught. I would stay curled up on the rug with Fluffett tucked warmly against my chest, listening to her rapid heartbeat. Bunnies' hearts can beat up to three hundred times per minute. Her twittering nose and fluttering whiskers would tickle my neck like a bird's feather, delighting me beyond imagination. When it was time to get up, it didn't seem so difficult with my little furry companion in my arms.

Could life with Fluffett open me up to an avenue of pain relief I had yet to explore?

Chapter 8

One day, Julie and Chris managed to persuade me to take Fluffett outside, though I wasn't easily sold. I had been stretched out on the couch in the sunroom beneath the ceiling fans that hot summer day, enriching my mind with Richard Adams's *Watership Down*, the ultimate read for the most passionate bunny lover. The unique, beautifully descriptive narrative is told from the point of view of a warren of rabbits in Down's England, documenting their reaction to mankind's encroachment onto their lifelong turf. I was picturing with great detail the hilarious, and sometimes perilous, journey the bunnies took through foreign landscapes as they tried to burrow their way to safety when Chris came up behind me.

"I want to take Fluffett outside, Mom. Jessica has an indoor rabbit that plays outside," said Chris, referring to our new babysitter.

"I am not sure that's a good idea, Chris."

Then he said it. "Mom, you're being irrational."

I ignored the false accusation, determined to remain rational. I had never considered bringing our bunny outside; we had bears and foxes in the neighborhood. Plus, I feared Fluffett might take off and get lost. But I hesitated too long, and Chris scooped Fluffett up. I yelled for Julie, the more cautious child, for help, but who was I kidding? She flew down the stairs and out the back door to help her brother! Soon, we were all gathered in the backyard.

Once set down on the grass, Fluffett immediately sat back on her haunches. A gentle breeze ruffled her fur as she gazed off into the distance. She looked exquisite in her natural environment of vast, soft greenery.

Fluffett turned her head slowly clockwise, then counterclockwise. Her pink nose was twittering faster than usual, and her eyes had an intensity about them. She was on high alert, observing a world full of edible greenery and underground warrens. *And dangerous animals,* I thought, worried. I was ready to leap should she make a run for it.

Once Fluffett had checked out her surroundings to her satisfaction, she ducked her head down and started sniffing the grass. It didn't take her long to figure out that the mass of green was not only soft and cozy but also delicious. She began nibbling the tips of the blades with the enthusiasm of a wild rabbit. It was beautiful to watch. Her molars went into overdrive, trimming a small patch of the lawn, until it struck me that the chemicals and fertilizers could be dangerous. I clapped my hands to distract her, inadvertently igniting an outdoor version of the Bunny Game. Fluffett popped up and tore across the lawn toward the woods.

"Split up and surround her," I yelled, looking frantically in every direction. I didn't want to frighten her by running after her and screaming. Fluffett circled two massive oak trees, crisscrossing the lawn and carving out figure eights in the grass.

"Where's the bunny?" I asked as I approached her, pretending that I, too, was playing the game. Then she spotted the elaborate, colorful swing set Ward had built from scratch for Julie and Chris. She stopped and chinned the wooden posts, which gave us enough time to circle her. She scaled the plastic slide halfway—impressively—then slid down backwards on her belly, landing on the grass in a small heap. She rolled over and started shimmying, her back paws bench pressing as if to say, "Oh yeah, this is where I'm supposed to be."

Chris dove next to her and did his own version of the "shake." They were so cute that I wanted to smother them both with kisses. I laid on the ground and wrapped my body around Chris and Fluffett, forming a cocoon, but she rolled back up on all fours and popcorned high into the air over our manmade enclosure and twirled across the grass, changing directions several times.

Julie threw a small ball from our bocce ball set across the lawn, yelling, "Get the ball, Fluffett!"

"She's not a golden retriever," said Chris sarcastically. "She's a bunny. You might try tossing a carrot, Jules."

"She's just as much fun as any dog," I exclaimed, "and a whole lot less work."

Chris shot me his "every boy needs a dog expression," followed by a half-smile.

Suddenly, a squirrel came crawling down the trunk of one of the nearby oak trees. We all saw it at the same time. A loud hissing frightened me. Fluffett stopped popcorning and lunged angrily toward the tree. She made a grunting sound as the squirrel crept further down along the thick moss. We had never heard her make such a noise. She charged again, head down, placing her front paws on the protruding roots of the oak tree, grunting and baring her teeth. Then she sat up and thumped. The noise sounded like a bowling ball dropping. Was she challenging the squirrel? The hissing intensified. I told the children to step back. The squirrel whipped its tail violently, smacking the tree trunk, and came within feet of Fluffett—close enough to scare her to near death. At least, that's what I had thought. Fluffett flipped her hind legs to retreat and landed on the grass in a seated position, where she remained. Her body was eerily still and appeared frozen. Her gaze was empty.

"Fluffett!" I shrieked. There was not a flutter of a whisker or wiggle of a nose. I presumed she had had a heart attack. I whisked her up and held her stiff body. I thought I might get sick. The muscles beneath her beautiful fur felt like a taut bicep. Her thumper legs were frozen at a ninety-degree angle to her body, and her front paws were curled like she was begging for food. "I think she had a heart attack," I screamed, feeling the blood rush to my extremities as I went into fight-or-flight mode. Julie was ready to burst into tears, but Chris, strangely, remained calm.

"It's a bunny survival technique," he said, with the assurance of someone who knew bunnies and all of their intricacies. "Fluffett's playing dead,"

"What?" It was all I was able to utter as fear overcame me.

"I read about it on one of the bunny websites. It's meant to fool a predator, Mom. I promise."

Could he possibly be right?

"God, please protect our bunny," I begged under my breath as I sat on the swing set, stroking Fluffett's stiff body, hoping somehow that I could transfer some of the life from my body to hers. Chris rushed over to comfort me, realizing I wasn't convinced. I was certain she had died. Thoughts of my childhood puppy Flop's death flooded my mind. I was completely overwhelmed—until I began to feel a strange sensation in Fluffett. Ever so slowly, life returned to her small, furry body.

I was never so happy to learn that Chris was indeed well-informed. We would later witness this bunny survival technique one more time in Fluffett's life.

"You scared us to death, Fluffett."

Once Julie and I calmed down, I walked toward the house with Fluffett. Outdoor playtime was over, as far as I was concerned. Suddenly, Fluffett's confidence seemed to return and she scratched my chest playfully, struggling to get free for another round of "Let's fool the enemy." Only the squirrel was now gone; my screams had sent him deep into the woods.

Chris grabbed her out of my arms and threw her back into play mode. She binkied along the grass near the sidewalk, then spotted in her peripheral vision a golf ball–sized hole in the dirt near the back porch. She scurried over and started digging with her front paws—left, right, left, right. Dirt flew up into the air, creating a small brown cloud. Within minutes, she had practically disappeared down the hole, giving me another adrenaline rush. Her tail was the only thing left sticking out above the ground.

"That's it," I screeched, yanking her tail lightly. "I think we've had enough of the great outdoors."

Fluffett attempted the great escape, yanking herself away from my grasp and taking a nosedive. My hands clutched her hips while she hung onto a cluster of grass with her front paws and teeth. She did the perfect handstand, putting up a good fight, but lost. I slung her on my chest and brushed off the loose dirt.

"You're an indoor bunny, Fluffett, and that's the law of the land," I announced as she darted up my shoulder and stared at the backyard pathetically, like a child being dragged into a time-out.

"Don't worry, Fluffett," said Chris. "I'll take you out again when she's not around."

My head spun around like one of those ventriloquist dolls. "What did you say, Chris?"

"I told Fluffett I'll take her out again sometime," he said indignantly.

Venom spewed from my breath. "If anything happens to this rabbit, you better start running and don't look back. I mean it."

"We know you mean it, Mom." Julie and Chris laughed together. "That's the scary part."

"You better be scared," I said, doing a bit of acting at this point, of course!

"What about all of the dirt?" Julie asked. Fluffett was licking herself profusely. Her once-pink tongue looked like beef jerky. "She's filthy."

"Let's give her a bath, kids."

"She'd lick herself clean in the wild," Chris retorted, but I wasn't listening. I was imagining streams of mud creeping through Fluffett's intestines and dirt strewn all over the house.

Julie ran upstairs and came back with an old hooded baby towel and her favorite Bath and Body Works shower gel, Cotton Candy. Climbing up and down the steps too often in a day can exacerbate my leg and back pain, so I was happy for Julie's help. Sometimes my arms and legs felt so heavy it seemed they were tied to cement blocks, and the smallest movement took effort. But I was determined to clean Fluffett. We filled the kitchen sink halfway with warm water, and I spread out clean dishtowels on the counter. Chris looked on disapprovingly.

Slowly, I lowered Fluffett's hind legs into the water first, holding her torso firmly under her armpits. She went ballistic, making the squirrel episode look tame. Her head swung backwards and her hind legs thumped against the side of the sink, splashing water everywhere. I struggled to hold onto her slippery body while Julie, under my guidance, quickly squeezed some shower gel onto her underside, which resembled a sandpit instead of a pile of cotton.

"Use the sprayer to rinse her, but gently," I managed to say. "Quickly!" My main focus was keeping Fluffett from thrashing too much and injuring herself. As the soap and water washed away the dirt and flowed down along her scut (the area beneath a bunny's tail), we stared at her underside and shrieked in disbelief. Little bunny foo foo was not a foo foo at all. Fluffett's male anatomy had been buried underneath thick, snow-white fur. It was impossible to imagine how we had missed it. Fluffett was a boy.

Julie and I started moping. Chris mimed doing the hula. The men would have the upper hand in the house, now.

"We'll have to change her name, kids." I felt a sense of excitement mounting over picking a more appealing name.

"I still like Fluffett," Julie replied in a solemn tone, clearly disappointed with our discovery.

"But Fluffett does not sound appropriate for a boy. I like the name Bunny Boy." I was ready to put up a good fight. No male pet of mine would have a name like Fluffett.

"But we like Fluffett."

"Who cleans the cage and feeds the bunny?" I joked, desperate for some leverage.

"We can call him both names," they replied.

"Precisely." I pulled back the hood of the towel and kissed our male bunny's ears.

And so, Bunny Boy went on record as the official name for our red satin rabbit.

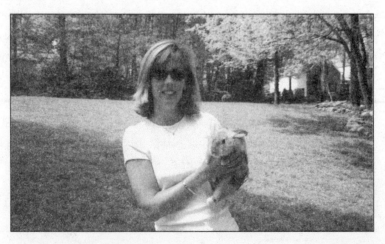

Chapter 9

Bunny Boy, as we now called him, was utterly lovable, spoiled, and demanding. My affection for him grew with each passing day. I found his quirky demands simply enchanting. If I drank my morning coffee before he had his slice of apple, he would thump loudly. If I sat down to read the newspaper or to answer some emails when he was in the mood to cuddle, he would dive at my ankles and nibble my toes until I picked him up. He had an endless supply of colorful and tasty chewable treats to satisfy any bunny's appetite, as well as plenty of toys, which he left all over the house. I had already been accused by my family of favoring him.

Bunny Boy seemed to adjust nicely to the whole gender and name change, but it took me some time. I had yet to come up with the right tune to sing to him when he plumped in his litter pan. I spent more than sufficient time practicing, "How's my boy?" giving special attention to tone, pitch, and inflection.

One morning, I walked downstairs with noticeably more spring in my steps, which, according to my family, was the new norm since Bunny Boy. He was lying on his side in the corner of his cage. He looked so peaceful. I noticed a flutter in my stomach—almost childlike.

"How's my boy?" I said, reaching down to pet his head. "Did you sleep well, little man?"

"She doesn't talk to us that way, does she Chris?" I overheard Julie say teasingly from the family room upstairs.

"Not to Dad, either," Chris replied.

Bunny Boy rolled over on all fours as if his body was too heavy to turn. Instead of charging out when he saw me, he hopped out of this cage slowly, painfully. His big ears were lying flat on top of his head—not erect like antennas as they usually were—and his jet-black eyes were translucent. He nudged my bare foot with his nose and just sat there instead of climbing up my shin. I picked him up, puzzled. His nose wasn't moist, and it was barely twittering. His food bowl looked untouched, and there were only a few pellets in his litter pan instead of the usual large pile.

"There's something wrong with Bunny Boy!" I yelled, with a sense of fear I somehow knew was warranted. Julie and Chris leapt down the stairs two at a time. I flipped through the yellow pages anxiously and found a veterinarian in Franklin Lakes.

We raced through the vet's door, past a dozen or more pets and their owners. Business seemed to be thriving. Bunny Boy laid on my chest with his chin on my shoulder while I filled out the paperwork. The receptionist looked at me quizzically; I wasn't sure why. The office was spacious and cheerful. In the lobby, a large tropical fish tank was placed against the far wall and bookcases were stocked with pet books and various supplies. Alongside the reception desk were half a dozen cages full of rescue kittens.

A technician named Kelly led us to an examination room down the hallway. I looked around at the diplomas hanging on the pale-green walls.

"No wonder the lobby was so crowded, Bunny Boy," I whispered. The veterinarian was a graduate of Cornell University, an Ivy League school in the northeast, and she had done her internship at the University of Pennsylvania, another Ivy League member. "Now we just need a good bedside manner, buddy."

Moments later, the door opened. An attractive young woman with a distinct air of confidence walked in and introduced herself. She didn't look much older than thirty-five.

"Hi, I'm Doctor Cheryl Welch," she said warmly. "So, tell me what's going on with Bunny Boy." Her casualness was refreshing.

"I don't think Bunny Boy has eaten or pooped in over twelve hours, and he's very listless. And his nose is dry and still. His whiskers aren't fluttering . . ." I was rambling. I pulled Bunny Boy closer to me, fearful for what could be wrong.

"Is that so, buddy?" she asked, gently petting Bunny Boy's head while looking immediately at his nose. "If you don't mind, Mrs. Laracy, I'd like to have an assistant come in and help while I examine Bunny Boy. Some bunnies bite or scratch when they're being examined. Or even thump. And the force of their hind legs could break your nose."

While it was hard for me to imagine Bunny Boy breaking anyone's nose, I responded, "Of course."

Kelly returned and gently restrained Bunny Boy around his torso while Dr. Welch examined his eyes, nose, ears, and mouth thoroughly with a lighted scope. She listened to his heart and lungs with her stethoscope and then his intestines twice. But for an occasional swipe at the scopes, Bunny Boy behaved remarkably.

"Is he always this calm and sweet?" asked Dr. Welch.

I thought back to the day when he went postal during his first bath.

"He is," I said, tongue-in-cheek.

"Bunny Boy most likely has a blockage in his gastrointestinal tract," she said matter-of-factly. "Bunnies must have food passing through their intestines at all times or their GI tract shuts down quickly, causing a condition known as gut stasis. They can die within thirty-six hours. How long did you say it has been since he last ate?"

"Twelve hours, right Mom?" said Julie.

Did she say die? I counted the hours in my head, trying to figure out the last time I had seen Bunny Boy eat or graze.

"Could Bunny Boy have eaten something in the house that he shouldn't have or has he had any new chew toys?"

"New toys?" said Chris. "Bunny Boy has the newest, most innovative chew toys on the market."

Dr. Welch flashed him a smile. "I bet he does."

I pictured Bunny Boy's fluorescent-colored wooden chew sticks shredded and stacked in the corner of his cage like a pile of colorful timber and wondered if they were the culprit.

"We'll use a drug called Propulsid to help Bunny Boy's gastrointestinal tract push along anything that could be causing the blockage," said Dr. Welch. I recognized the name—I, too, had taken the drug once for reflux.

"What about giving him syrup of ipecac to get him to throw up whatever could be causing the blockage?" I asked.

"Bunnies have a one-way esophagus and cannot throw up," she explained. "Our safest and best bet is the Propulsid. If that doesn't work, the other option would be surgery, but the postoperative mortality rate among rabbits is extremely high."

She spoke in a manner that conveyed the intelligence and experience of someone older. But I was stunned. Surgery? Mortality rate?

"Rabbits can be frail creatures, I am afraid to say," Dr. Welch remarked. "They succumb to pain and discomfort quickly. They also hide their ailments very well. Often until it is too late. But I think we caught this early enough. I do."

"More than dogs or cats?"

"For sure." She wrapped her arm around my shoulder with the tenderness you would receive from a dear friend, not a veterinarian you had just met. She was lovely.

"I'd like you to give Bunny Boy some pineapple juice in a dropper and baby food—carrots—to help soften his stools. You may have to force-feed him."

Force-feed a member of the Food Family?

"Hopefully you should start to see half-formed fecal pellets, then full-size pellets within the next day or so. If Bunny Boy gets more than a little diarrhea, call me immediately. We run a slippery slope. Too much diarrhea can be dangerous."

What's more than a little? I thought. I glanced over at the kids. They were speechless, a rare occurrence.

Dr. Welch made some final notations in Bunny Boy's chart and weighed him. He was four pounds, nine ounces, much more than I would have expected.

"Is Bunny Boy fully grown?" I asked.

"He's only eight months old, is that correct?"

"Yes. He was born in December."

"Bunny Boy's peak weight should be about nine pounds, give or take. He won't reach that until he's well over a year old."

"Nine pounds? That's impossible," I exclaimed. "They said he was a dwarf."

"Who told you that?"

I shook my head. "The same person who told us he was a girl."

"Maybe a dwarf elephant!" she laughed, strumming Bunny Boy's ears happily through her fingers. "Bunny Boy's a red satin, and he's going to be a big boy."

I'm not sure how we had missed that critical fact on the Internet. We were certainly learning hilarious, and some harrowing, things by trial and error. Finally, Chris was able to muster up some positive emotion to break the silence.

"If I can't have a big dog, at least I'll have a big rabbit."

In the car ride to the supermarket, Bunny Boy laid on his side on the backseat between Julie and Chris, barely moving. As I scanned the aisles searching for baby food, carrots, and pineapple juice, a rush of emotions hit me like a ton of bricks. I wandered over to the checkout line like a lost soul. My cell phone buzzed. It was Ward.

"I'm not sure," I mumbled, feigning poor cell phone reception when he asked how much I had spent at the veterinarian. "What does it matter anyway?"

The ten-minute ride home seemed interminable. Conversation was limited. We gave new meaning to the phrase *gloom and doom*. Tenderly, Julie carried Bunny Boy into the house and placed him in his litter pan. He loved the comfort of the soft pine shavings. He crouched down and closed his eyes. We had never seen him close his eyes completely before. When he napped, they were always half open. Any remaining battery juice in his body seemed to be dwindling. It was scary.

I offered to make breakfast, but nobody was hungry. So we organized Bunny Boy's medicine and food.

"The drugs are crushed. The instruments are sterile," I said as I worked, trying to lighten the mood.

"The pineapple juice is ready," Chris mimicked.

Julie sat Bunny Boy on her lap while I lowered the spoon of carrots and crushed Propulsid toward his mouth. His tongue thrust forward quickly, like a rattlesnake, lapping up the carrots and catching us by surprise.

"Bunny Boy likes it!" she exclaimed. Chris grabbed the spoon out of my hand and took his turn, bringing it toward Bunny Boy's mouth like an airplane. I managed to chuckle, remembering my days of using the same tactic to get Chris to eat baby cereal. Bunny Boy lapped up the second spoon, and suddenly he was up on all fours, licking his chops with great satisfaction. I released the syringe of pineapple juice into the corner of his mouth and his tongue flicked from side to side, savoring every drop. He clearly loved the new menu. In a moment of weakness and relief, I promised Bunny Boy that I would put away his cage and that he could roam free at night if he would start going to the bathroom.

"We can't live without you buddy," Chris whispered in Bunny Boy's flat ears. "We love you."

Life without Bunny Boy? I refused to let the possibility enter my mind. Everything was going to be fine, wasn't it?

By midafternoon, Bunny Boy still had not gone to the bathroom. It was unnerving. I would have welcomed a big brown pile of poop with open arms. We fed him again, and he ate with the same enthusiasm, but when he finished he quickly fell back to sleep.

It was nearly dinnertime when Bunny Boy sat up in his litter pan and maneuvered into his favorite position to take a dump. Fifteen tense minutes passed. Then twenty. I couldn't wait any longer. I lifted him off of his litter pan as he resisted. Miraculously, I had interrupted his long-awaited bowel movement. The kids and I joined arms and swung around in a circle, celebrating the pile of half formed pellets.

By morning, Bunny Boy had eaten a humongous pile of hay and filled his litter pan with enough "full-size capers" to supply an Italian bistro.

Thankfully, Bunny Boy had dodged the first bullet. We had survived the first of many medical crises that were yet to come.

Chapter 10

As I already knew all too well, life is unpredictable and scary. And you always seem to be reminded of it when you're settling down to cuddle with your favorite bunny or loved one. I was sitting in the sunroom with Bunny Boy tucked under my arm and a newspaper in the other, the warmth of my rabbit radiating across my lap, when the phone rang. Ward brought it to me. I could tell by the look on his face that it wasn't good.

"It's your brother, Tom."

I could hear the anguish in Tom's voice. Unconsciously, I hugged Bunny Boy tighter. "It's Audrey," Tom said, choking back the tears. Bunny Boy became very still, as if he were waiting along with me for the bad news. "She's got stage three thyroid cancer. She needs to have surgery immediately. We are going to need some help, Nance. Can you come to Denver?"

My heart immediately leapt to my throat. Tom's wife, Audrey, was only thirty-eight years old and their boys, the "Irish twins" of the family, were just four and five. How could this be happening? Suddenly, I realized I was standing, though I didn't remember getting up. The newspaper I had been reading was scattered on the floor by my feet. Somehow, Bunny Boy was still tucked under my arm, holding on for dear life. I put down the phone and stroked Bunny Boy's soft ears while Ward purchased a flight on the Internet.

I gazed through the wall of windows and past the tall trees, dismissing their beauty. "I'm so sad, Bunny Boy," I said. He nuzzled closer, as if he understood. I suddenly thought of Flop and realized that her compassionate spirit had somehow been reincarnated into a red satin rabbit. How had I ever lived without this bunny in my life?

I called my mother and found her in tears. Tom had called her first. She had nursed Tommy back to health when he was a sick child with an intensity that only a mother can muster, and their special bond persevered after he got well. Tom was her baby, the only one of her children who had inherited her black hair and dark brown eyes.

My mother and I made plans to fly out the next evening. Mom had had back surgery three weeks prior, but in true Mom fashion she insisted on making the trip for her son and daughter-in-law. That night, I found my rosary beads in their usual spot—under my bed pillow—and I prayed fervently while Bunny Boy purred softly beside me, doing his bunny best to comfort me.

The next morning, Bunny Boy pranced out from under the dining room chair, wide-eyed and bushy tailed, as if trying to convince me that today was a new day, reason enough to celebrate life. I tried to disguise my sadness and the fact that my joints and muscles were aching due to a stress-induced flare-up. "Where's my boy, and what did you do?" I said in my best cheerful voice.

Bunny Boy picked up his stride and tore across the oriental rug when he heard me. He tripped on the fringe and slid across the kitchen tile, plunging into the cabinet that housed overcrowded pots and pans. The door flew open and a barrage of Teflon came crashing to the floor, nearly hitting him. But Bunny Boy was too fast. Using the force of his back legs, he sent one of the smaller pots sailing across the floor and swatted another with his front paws, flipping it upside down and right side up. Then he sat in it and peed. I was shocked. I snuck up behind Bunny Boy and crouched down to his level, looking right into his eyes. "Where's my boy, and what did you do?" I repeated, trying my hardest to be mad at him but not quite managing. Bunny Boy wrapped his little front paws around my knees gingerly and stretched his head up to kiss me. His brand of bunny therapy worked like a charm. For ten seconds, I had forgotten all about my brother and Audrey. But then another thought hit me. I was going to have to leave Ward in charge of both the kids *and* the bunny. How was he going to handle that with his schedule?

I called our tennis and swim club and enrolled Julie and Chris in the day camp so they would be supervised while Ward was at work. I phoned Ward at work with the update. He assured me again that he would work shorter hours and take "impeccable" care of Bunny Boy and the children. I knew he would, but I went over the instructions for Bunny Boy's care numerous times, just to be sure. Ward made no attempt to mask his sigh on the other end of the line. I could hear him using his calculator while I rambled.

"Repeat the instructions back to me, honey," I said, not satisfied that he had memorized them. The phone clicked. I hit speed dial. I knew the kids could fend for themselves if need be, but with Bunny Boy, I wasn't taking any chances.

My mother and I arrived in Denver around two-thirty in the morning. We drove into the blackness, past the bright white caps of the airport building's terminals and heading for the real peaks. Mom was rattling off directions from MapQuest like she had drunk ten cups of coffee.

"You're a real trooper, Mom." I whispered. "We're all so lucky to have you."

•   •   •

My mother smiled and her eyes twinkled. "I'm the one who's lucky, sweetheart. Don't ever forget that." I knew that I never would. I felt the same way about my children, and I hoped they'd always remember that, too.

When we pulled into the driveway, I could see Tom's silhouette through the picture window in the front of the house. The three of us embraced the moment we walked through the door and shed enough tears to start a mudslide.

"Thank god you're here," Tom said when we finally let go of each other. "I've been sitting here trying to make some sense of this nightmare. It doesn't seem possible. Why is this happening, Mom?"

"Your sister and I will help you work through some of this. God will do the rest," said my mother. Her unshakable faith had gotten us all through my brother's illness and my father's heart attacks.

I descended into the man cave in the basement at four in the morning and literally fell onto the futon out of sheer exhaustion. I was in overwhelming pain from the traveling—handling the luggage and pushing my mother, who was still recovering from back surgery, in a wheelchair through the airport—and I quickly felt ashamed for even thinking about my pain during such a terrible time for Tom and Audrey. Briefly, I thought of Bunny Boy and tried to imagine him curled up on my chest, wiggling his nose. Eventually, I fell asleep.

In what felt like ten minutes later, eight pounds of male dog pounced on my chest, waking me from a troubled rest. It was seven a.m.

"No, Jake!" Tom's boys, Evan and Drew, jumped on top of me along with the dog, nearly squeezing the breath out of my body. The boys were identical in size, despite being a year apart in age, and very handsome. Drew resembled his mother—light hair, fair skin. Evan was a clone of his father—thick black hair and olive skin.

We climbed up the stairs—one nephew under each arm and Jake at my heels. My mother and Tom were sitting in front of the bay window that overlooked the foothills of the Rocky Mountains. The backdrop was spectacular. The tall, jagged mountain peaks cut into the blue sky, and there were small clusters of white clouds as far as the eye could see. A dark cloud hovered above the tallest peak, dropping snowflakes even though it was summer. The sun bathed the entire back of the house. "We put our sunglasses on before our slippers out here," said Tom. I spotted a wild bunny deep in the greenery and pictured Bunny Boy many miles away, munching on his lettuce.

I started breakfast for the boys, helping to keep a semblance of normalcy in a household that had been rocked to its core. Audrey walked into the kitchen. She looked sweet but pale, her strawberry blonde curls falling just above her shoulders. Her faded jeans hugged her curves. I held her close. I could feel her body trembling. "Thank you for coming," said Audrey, whose soothing voice always sounded like a meandering stream.

We drove north along the base of the Rocky Mountains. The sound of the diesel engine broke the silence. What could we say? I desperately wanted to tell Audrey that everything was going to be fine, but I didn't know for sure. The road ahead could be long and difficult. So, we rode in silence into an unpredictable future of whatever was going to happen next. And no matter what happened, we knew we would face it together, as we always did.

The look of fear on Audrey's face as they brought her into the operating room was haunting. I couldn't get it out of my mind. Nine and a half hours later, the surgeon walked into the waiting area, his face drawn and dotted with perspiration.

"The tumor was encapsulated," he said and patted my brother on the back with an exhausted surgeon's reassuring smile. "I think we got it all." Tom broke down and sobbed in my arms.

Seeing Audrey was devastating at first. A macabre necklace of stitches ran from one ear across her throat to the other, which I quickly realized would become a badge of honor for this young woman—a mother and wife, my sister, and a good friend—who was going to beat the cancer with her usual quiet strength and determination.

Before any of us had a chance to catch our breath and rejoice, the second wave crashed onto the shore. The next morning, my phone started ringing at the alarmingly early hour of six a.m. I rummaged through my purse in the dark, half asleep. It was only eight in the morning at home. What could have happened?

It was Ward. "What's up honey?" I asked. "Do you miss me?" We had never been apart from each other for more than a weekend since we married, and neither one of us liked to be separated for long.

"It's Bunny Boy," Ward said. I could tell by the sound of his voice that he had been afraid to call me with the news. "He's got a growth the size of a tennis ball hanging from his chin."

I bolted upright in the futon. "And you just noticed it?" I said, sounding a bit more accusatory than I meant to.

"It wasn't there when I spoke to you last night," said Ward helplessly.

"Does Bunny Boy seem to be in pain?"

"I found him sitting hunched over from the weight of the thing. It can't be comfortable."

I sprang into action. It was Sunday morning and Dr. Welch wasn't in. I called home to my sister, Carol, and got the name of a twenty-four-hour veterinarian. I called Ward back.

"Please take Bunny Boy to the vet immediately and call me when you get there." Then, I paced the man cave anxiously, waiting for the phone to ring. I had never anticipated such worrisome medical problems with Bunny Boy.

Though my trip to Denver was on short notice, I thought I had done a stellar job covering all the bases. I had left no stone unturned in my preparations for any eventuality. The refrigerator was stocked and there was a bale of hay and six heads of romaine lettuce for Bunny Boy. Post-its hung on all visible surfaces in the kitchen, and large, colorful signs were taped on each door leading outside—"Don't do it. Mom will kill you." I had reorganized the drug drawer, moving my prescriptions to the left and keeping benign items like Tylenol, Pepto-Bismol, and cough syrup in the basket to the right, marked with more Post-its—"Stomach aches only. Not dessert. Sweating doesn't count." As a joke, I had taped Dr. Welch's phone number to the headboard to our bed, but I had never in a million years thought that Ward would need to use it.

My mother was mixing batter for pancakes when "Moon River," my ringtone of choice, finally played on my cell phone. When I picked it up, all I could hear in the background was a terrible, high-pitched, relentless shrilling. I knew it was Bunny Boy. It was the most horrible, terrifying sound I had ever heard. I finally understood why the sharpshooters at Waco, Texas, used audio recordings of terrified rabbits to lure out hostage takers. "Bunny Boy had a huge abscess on his jaw," said Ward calmly, trying to head off my clear distress. "The technician put him in a headlock while the doctor squeezed the thing like it was a huge pimple right in front of us. It was horrible."

I instantly felt nauseous. My adrenaline kicked in. What if Bunny Boy died of a heart attack from fear or pain? Rabbits have weak hearts . . .

"Thank god you weren't here," added Ward, trying to tease me. "You'd be on trial for murder." With Ward, legal references of one sort or another always cropped up no matter the circumstance. I tried to block out the screaming. *It's an abscess, and Ward has it under control*, I told myself. But then I heard the sound of Chris crying.

"Why is Chris crying?" I asked, and Ward hesitated. "Ward?"

"There's no cure for these types of abscesses, Nancy."

"But that's impossible," I said, trying to compose myself. What was he talking about?

"I can't be alone with Julie and Chris if this rabbit dies," Ward said. "Is there any way you might be able to come home tonight instead of tomorrow night?"

"Tonight? I don't know, Ward. How can I leave Audrey?" I said. "I need to think this through. I'll talk to Tom and call you back." As soon as I hung up, Tom came down the stairs and put his arm around me.

"We'll be just fine; we're out of the woods now, Nance," he said. He nodded his head yes and smiled when he saw my uncertainty. "You need to be with them. They need you now. Animals are like a member of the family." Tom looked over at Jake, who was curled up on Drew's lap. I knew my brother understood, but I needed to talk to Audrey before I made my decision.

I sat by Audrey on the sofa shortly after dusk and we talked—easily, happily, the way we always do. She was so brave. I thought how lucky we all were that, at least for now, our wonderful Audrey was safe. She reassured me that the worst was over and that they would be all right without us. Thankfully, their church and neighborhood had organized childcare and meals for the next three weeks. She thanked me again for coming and told me she loved me. Still, despite her reassurances, I walked into the kitchen with great trepidation and heaviness, wondering if I was making the right decision, and called Ward. I told him I was coming home.

I knew some people would think I was crazy to leave my sister-in-law to rush home to Bunny Boy, but something told me I needed to do it. If only I had known then how my decision to come home early would come to profoundly affect the rest of my life.

Once again, my poor mother and I boarded a plane on a moment's notice, taking the red-eye and heading home. A driver was waiting for us outside the departure hall, holding a sign that read "Laracy"—written inside the outline of a bunny. I forced a smile.

My hands shook as I punched in the code to the garage door. The house was eerily quiet. As the cage came into view, I saw Bunny Boy sitting on his haunches in his litter pan. The abscess was painfully visible. I rushed over and picked him up gently. "How's my little boy?" I said, nearly choking on my words. He looked sad and beat-up. I kissed his droopy ears and sweet little paws, nuzzling him deep in my neck. His nose was dry. His whiskers were at a standstill.

"I'm home now," I whispered. "Mommy's home." Then I felt it. The subtle fluttering of his whiskers. Bunny Boy started to purr.

When I looked up, Ward was standing on the landing of the stairs. We wrapped our arms around each other, cradling Bunny Boy between us, feeling the warmth of his small body, grateful to be together again.

Then I peeked in quietly on Julie and Chris in their beds. I had missed them so much. Julie looked peaceful, curled up in her crowded bed full of lime-green pillows and Beanbo, her old, faded-pink stuffed rabbit. Beanbo, which had arrived the day of her christening wrapped in pink cellophane and tied with a large pink bow, was her lifelong blankie. Chris was asleep on top of his plaid comforter, covered in sweat as usual. He seemed to have been born with a faulty internal thermostat. I breathed a sigh of relief to see both kids sleeping peacefully.

Today would be a difficult day. I was sure of it.

• • •

I phoned Dr. Welch's office and took an eleven o'clock appointment. Julie and Chris took a day off from school and came along. Nobody had gotten much sleep the night before.

The veterinarian's office was packed again, standing room only. A rainbow-colored bird that was propped on his owner's shoulder piqued my interest—and Bunny Boy's. The bird was peering down into a carrier that housed a beautiful cat with long black hair and emerald green eyes. It uttered a variety of sounds that ranged in volume—all of which had special meaning, according to her proud owner. All of which startled Bunny Boy. He clawed his way up my chest, hanging onto me for dear life.

When we were finally called into the office, Dr. Welch cupped Bunny Boy's head and examined the abscess. Despite being drained at the emergency vet, it had grown to the size of a golf ball again. Chris couldn't help himself. He blurted out the grizzly details of their visit the night before.

"I'm sorry you had to go through that, honey," said Dr. Welch, gently pushing the hair back on his forehead. She had a beautiful way about her and an infectious smile. She examined the inside of Bunny Boy's mouth thoroughly. "The abscess stems from the root of his tooth," She explained, remarking that his teeth were misaligned—a malocclusion. "Bunny Boy could use some braces," she said, winking at Chris.

Then she looked at me and became more serious. "These abscesses are common in bunnies and almost impossible to cure," she said. I saw a glint of moisture in Chris's eyes. "Hay works well as dental floss for rabbits, but it can also puncture their gums, allowing bacteria to enter. In a healthy rabbit, it's not usually a problem, but more than likely, Bunny Boy was born with a compromised immune system. I'll need to draw some blood."

I couldn't believe what I was hearing. Did she just say that Bunny Boy might have a compromised immune system? How was it possible that I had adopted a rabbit that had similar autoimmune problems I did, and ones that were just as incurable? This was crazy.

"If we can keep the infection out of his organs or bloodstream for six months, we'll be lucky." Dr. Welch added sadly.

"But he's just a baby! What about surgery?" I said, with the same blind determination that had characterized my reaction to my own incurable condition. I had refused to accept defeat for myself, and I certainly wasn't going to accept defeat for Bunny Boy.

"Debriding an abscess is fairly routine with humans or other mammals, but the anesthesia poses a much greater risk for a rabbit. Their hearts are weak," she explained.

"Will Bunny Boy die soon without the surgery?" I asked. Dr. Welch didn't answer me, but she patted my arm gently, the way she had brushed back my son's hair. That said it all.

"I want him to have a chance at a full life," I said, fighting back the tears.

"Of course. I understand. We can schedule the surgery for Thursday and see how he does, but I want you to prepare yourself for the possibility that we could lose him."

I refused once again to let thoughts of losing Bunny Boy enter my mind. I threw my arms around her without reservation, feeling thankful that she was willing to give Bunny Boy a chance. As Dr. Welch hugged me back tightly, I knew in an instant that Bunny Boy would be in the very best of hands. If anybody could help our bunny beat the odds, it was this remarkable doctor.

"One other thing: try applying some hot compresses to Bunny Boy's jaw. They'll make him more comfortable and soften the contents of the abscess. It will be easier to drain."

• • •

Julie and Chris had many questions on the short ride home. Questions I couldn't and didn't want to answer. I called Scuffy's, and Loretta gave me the name of another veterinarian in the area who worked with rabbits. I wanted to be sure we were doing the right thing. The prognosis was just as bleak, but I refused to accept it. Neither veterinarian knew whom they were dealing with. And neither did Bunny Boy—yet.

When I left the cardiac wing of a hospital six years ago in 1995 with a clear diagnosis of acute parvovirus B-19 and was told that there was no treatment for the virus, I did some research of my own. I found two published studies in the *New England Journal of Medicine* and the *Lancet* in which doctors in Europe experimented with the use of intravenous gamma globulin as a treatment for acute cases of parvovirus. The medical community was just beginning to fully discover the devastating effects of acute parvovirus in adults—and women in particular. Parvovirus, previously known at Fifth's disease, is, under most circumstances, a benign virus that usually strikes children, giving them mild cold symptoms, fever, and a distinct lace-looking rash on their extremities along with bright red cheeks. I immediately brought the studies to my rheumatologist who promptly tossed them and refused to consider the treatment. His ego couldn't take it. But I wasn't taking no for an answer.

The next day, I called the Center for Disease Control in Atlanta, Georgia, and they asked me to send them a sample of my blood. They were researching the prevalence of acute parvovirus B-19 cases in the United States. Within days of receiving my blood sample, they enrolled me in a study and found me a new rheumatologist in New Jersey named Dr. Debra Pasik who ran a more open-minded practice. I became a candidate to receive the cutting-edge treatment. After six months of IV gamma globulin treatment once a month, the virus stopped replicating in my DNA and ceased to wreak havoc on my body, but I was left with the damage it had done to my immune system in the form of a connective tissue disease and fibromyalgia. I also lived with the memories of the muscle cramps, fevers, and severe malaise that I endured during the treatments, along with the anxiety of the possibility that I could go into anaphylactic shock, which was one of the rarer but more serious side effects of that powerful medicine—which could be fatal.

I had demanded so much for my care. So why on earth would I settle for any less for Bunny Boy? Somehow, somewhere, we would find a way to fight this together. And because we were together, I knew we could beat the odds.

Twenty hot compresses and forty-eight hours later, the kids and I dropped Bunny Boy off for his surgery. We waited breathlessly together for the doctor's call. My mother came over to comfort us and pray. When Dr. Welch finally called, it was as if she sensed our dreadful anticipation, and she chimed right in with the good news.

"Bunny Boy did great," she warbled into the phone. I gave the thumbs up to the kids and my mother, and we all cheered spontaneously. The hot compresses had paid off. As if there hadn't been enough good news for one day, Tom called right after I hung up with Dr. Welch. Audrey's pathology had come back clean. The cancer hadn't metastasized. It was a terrific day.

My close friend Mary Beth brought me to pick Bunny Boy up that afternoon. During my many years upon this planet, I had learned that girlfriends play a vital role in your life, each at different times. Mary Beth had strong faith. She had been a source of tremendous inspiration during the earlier days of my illness and had also noticed how my pain, energy level, and attitude on life had improved since Bunny Boy's arrival. She already knew how much we needed each other.

I took one look at Bunny Boy, who was wrapped in a fleece blanket, and gasped. The fur on his neck had been shaved, and he had a necklace of stitches almost identical to Audrey's. Three similar tubes, like the ones Audrey had post-op, hung from the middle of the incision. It was eerie and shocking. The enormous boo-boo made him look especially tiny. When I held him, I was afraid I might hurt him.

"Keep Bunny Boy warm while the anesthesia wears off," Dr. Welch instructed. A hot water bottle was tucked inside the blanket. She handed me a bag. "He has had pain medication that should last twenty-four hours. Give him some of the critical care liquid food supplements that's in this bag in a few hours. Force-feed him if you have to. He also had his first penicillin injection. Bunny Boy will need them every other day for six weeks, along with an oral antibiotic. The instructions and supplies are also in the bag."

Dr. Welch ended her instructions with a smile. "Please bring him back the day after tomorrow, and we'll show you how to give him his shot."

I was unnerved. While I had given myself many injections of anti-viral drugs and B vitamins over the course of my own illness, I couldn't imagine giving Bunny Boy shots. I was too emotionally attached to him. I walked out in a daze.

What could have been a tense ride home turned into a sitcom. It was ninety-five degrees outside and the air conditioning wasn't on. With Bunny Boy and his hot water bottle on my lap, I broke into an intense sweat—like those people who voluntarily put themselves through hot yoga.

"Can we please put on the air conditioning?" I asked, trying not to sound impatient. Reluctantly, Mary Beth slowly turned up the dial. All of a sudden, a smelly, pink, milky substance splattered everywhere—all over my furry patient and me. In a frenzy, Mary Beth turned the dial back up by mistake. Bunny Boy licked one drop of the sweet stuff and scrambled to get out of his blanket. He teetered like the Pillsbury doughboy from the anesthesia, knocking his water bottle to the floor. The cap must have been loose, and water poured onto the rug. To top it off, he peed on the seat. In less than five minutes, the van was completely funkified—in Technicolor.

"One of my children spilled their strawberry milkshake down the air ducts this morning," said Mary Beth, laughing. "Never a dull moment with kids in the house."

For the rest of the afternoon, Bunny Boy wobbled around like a drunken pool player who had lost a fight. He went right back to thrashing magazines with his teeth, headbutting things in his path, and squeezing under the coffee tables. I was afraid he would rip out one of his tubes or the stitches. His face was black and blue, and his head had swollen to twice its normal size. He fit right in with the Laracy family—two separate prenatal ultrasounds on both our children three and a half years apart, two different technicians, and the comments were identical.

"I can see that big heads run in the family," each of them said, looking specifically at Ward.

Shortly after dinner, Bunny Boy tried to drink from his bottle. He moved his head in all sorts of contorted positions, then banged the metal tip with his head. With his swollen head, he couldn't maneuver into the right position to lick the ball. He took his frustrations out on the three tubes hanging from his neck. Though he was unsteady on his feet, there was nothing wrong with his eye-paw coordination. I intercepted immediately.

"Don't even think about touching those things," I said sternly. Bunny Boy swung at the tubes again, taunting me. I got down on the floor and put my face right up to his nose, repeating my threat like the nuns at Catholic grammar school used to do to me.

"Maybe Bunny Boy can drink from a bowl. He's a highly intelligent animal," teased Chris. Chris and I were still battling the same ongoing argument—that I thought bunnies were more intelligent than he did. Bunny Boy flipped the first bowl of water upside down and sloshed his front paws around in the water. I poured water into a heavier, shallower bowl, but he bumped it with his head and looked up at us when it didn't flip. Then, being the smart animal he was, Bunny Boy moved the tubes out of his way with his left paw and lapped up the water as if he were a dog or a cat. He was simply amazing.

I took advantage of the moment and filled a large syringe with his critical care food supplement. We tried wrapping a towel loosely around his neck as a bib, but he grabbed it with his front teeth and tossed it to the floor. I placed the tip of the syringe near his mouth, and he started sucking down the apple banana goop so fast it oozed out of the side of his mouth. He ate seven large syringes of food before he finally stopped. I was afraid he would explode. Covered in food, he looked like a green monster, the floor beneath him a swamp. But I was so excited to see him eating that I didn't give the mess a second thought.

We brought Bunny Boy's cage, which he no longer used, upstairs to my bedroom that night. I placed it within inches of my side of the bed, near the nightlight where I could watch him carefully. I successfully lured him into his safe haven with a new wicker toy and a spoon of melted yogurt drops.

"It's just for a few nights, pal. It's for your own safety," I said. Bunny Boy didn't look convinced. He paced his cage relentlessly that night and clawed at the top rungs, looking for an escape route. Ward resorted to sleeping with a pillow wrapped over his ears. Around two in the morning, I caught Bunny Boy swiping the tubes.

"Please don't touch the tubes, little buddy," I hissed, trying not to wake my finally sleeping husband. Defiantly, Bunny Boy whacked them again. I slung myself on top of the cage.

"What part of 'Don't touch those tubes or stitches' don't you understand?" I said, as if I were talking to the kids. Bunny Boy cowered in his litter pan and stared up at me, compliant. "Get some rest, Bunny Boy."

But of course, he didn't. Around four in the morning, Ward got up and went to sleep in the spare bedroom, mumbling what I think was something about a crepuscular animal, though it came out sounding a lot more like "crappy creature." After all, Bunny Boy was depriving him of a second night of sleep.

• • •

Bunny Boy turned out to be far more resilient than anybody anticipated—which, we would come to realize over time, was just his style. Within a couple of days, he was nibbling on his food pellets, grazing on his hay, and drinking from a bowl like he had never heard of the word *abscess*.

"He's drinking from a bowl?" Dr. Welch asked during his postsurgical check-up.

"Can you believe it?" I said, shaking my head.

She drew up a syringe of penicillin and effortlessly gave Bunny Boy his injection while I observed.

"Their skin is like leather, so use a dart-like motion when you give him his shot," she said. Still, I had serious doubts about my ability to give Bunny Boy any of his injections.

"How are you, Mrs. Laracy?" she suddenly said. "You look a little tired." Somehow, the moment felt right. I quickly told her of my own heart-wrenching medical journey and explained that I, like Bunny Boy, was wrestling with autoimmune disease.

"Women are very strong creatures, aren't we?" she said, smiling. I looked around at her thriving practice and her Ivy League credentials and the pictures of her children.

"Yes, we are," I said, meaning it.

"By the way, Bunny Boy's bloodwork was conclusive," said Dr. Welch. "He is immune-compromised."

"It's a little ironic that I bought a bunny with an immune system problem, don't you think?" I said.

She smiled. "Someone knew just where to put Bunny Boy, didn't they?"

"Yes, they did," I said. I knew that my dad who watched over me, and now Bunny Boy, too, probably had had a hand in this miraculous match-up.

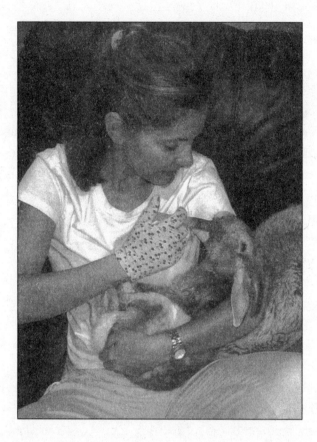

Chapter 11

Bunny Boy's delicate stature and my deep love for him made it too difficult for me to administer the shots of penicillin. My hands got sweaty and my body tensed up the first time I poked him. I was unsuccessful, leaving the milky-white substance trailing down his fur. Knowing how detail-oriented and methodical Ward was, I asked for his help. Ward was the epitome of quiet strength when situations required it.

"My billing rate is around three hundred and fifty dollars an hour, Nance," he said with a surly smile meant to relax me. I gave him one of my favorite looks, one he couldn't refuse.

Some shots went better than others. Every night around eight o' clock, I would hunt down Bunny Boy and place him on a freshly cleaned towel on the kitchen counter. I'd gently secure his hips, apologizing to him for what we were about to do, and Ward would gather up his scruff and give him the penicillin. Then, Bunny Boy got his rewards. A kiss from me. A hug from Ward. And a tiny piece of fruit. By the fifth shot, Bunny Boy barely seemed to notice.

Things were rolling along just fine in the house again. We only had one more week of shots left to do. I thought the worst was over. Then, one morning, I found Bunny Boy lying on the throw rug by the back door, covered in diarrhea. He looked like one of the animals in the BP oil commercials that had rolled in an oil slick. I sprinted to the phone and dialed Dr. Welch.

"Stop giving him the oral antibiotic and any food other than hay," she said with a sense of urgency that frightened me. "Give him some water in a syringe and lots of hay, and call me if Bunny Boy gets lethargic.

I will be in all day and will check back with you before I leave at four thirty."

I stood there, holding the phone away from my ear, thinking, *What's next?* Then I yelled up the stairs for help with the clean-up.

"You wanted that animal," Ward remarked. "Bathe him and lock him up in his cage, Nance. Let's keep the mess contained."

I let out a sigh of frustration. Ward was so logical, but I didn't want logical right now.

"I can't. I promised Bunny Boy that I would never lock him in his cage again."

Ward washed the kitchen floor and the unsightly brown mess that had marked the stairs and the family room. The kids—bribed with their favorite dessert, Black Bottom cupcakes—and I gave Bunny Boy a bath. He barely resisted when I placed him in the warm, sudsy water filled with lavender bubble bath. It worried me. With the air conditioning set at what felt like subzero temperatures in the house, we decided to blow-dry Bunny Boy's fur. The gentle humming of the blow-dryer on the lowest speed relaxed his tense body instead of startling him.

I spent the rest of the day quarantined in the kitchen with Bunny Boy, giving him periodic butt baths and taking any help I could get with clean-up duty. I refused to cage him, though I knew it would make my job easier. My bunny and I played and cuddled. I didn't care that he was dirty and smelly. For the rest of the day, Bunny Boy drank enthusiastically from his bowl and devoured his pile of hay as if nothing were wrong. As night fell, I made a makeshift bed out of some blankets and slept on the floor while my family abandoned me for the warmth of their beds. Being the crepuscular animal he was, Bunny Boy tore around the room like a cyclone, unfazed by his bowel problems. He scurried all over me while I longed for the softness of my bed. He nuzzled shamelessly in my neck, the peach fuzz around his incision tickling me. I hugged him tight and prayed. "It's just a little diarrhea, another bump in the road," I tried to convince myself.

I must have finally dozed off from sheer exhaustion, only to be woken by Julie's beautiful voice and smile.

"Mom, look!" she whispered.

I was lying on my side with my knees pulled up toward my chest. Bunny Boy was tucked into the small space between my chest and legs, so close to my heart that I could feel his breathing. I picked my head up and glanced backward over my hips and saw what Julie was referring to. There was a pile of pellets at the bottom of my blanket, but no diarrhea. In that moment, any pain I felt from sleeping on the floor seemed meaningless. I was ecstatic and relieved.

"I think Bunny Boy is going to be just fine, honey," I said, yawning, and returned to my fetal position.

Chapter 12

"My CRP level is seventeen?" I gasped.

I was on the phone with my rheumatologist, Dr. Pasik. I hung up, feeling temporarily beaten down. The creatine reactive protein (CRP) level in a healthy person is supposed to be zero. Seventeen was way out of the acceptable range, which meant there was significant inflammation throughout my body, despite my being on steroids for the past six weeks. And unfortunately, when my connective tissue disease flared up, the fibromyalgia usually did as well. It was a double whammy. Dealing with the different symptoms, medications, and underlying systemic issues of two diseases was not for the faint of heart.

Thankfully I did not suffer from depression or anxiety, which is often seen in fibromyalgia patients. Irritable bowel syndrome is another symptom that plagues fibromyalgia patients—and after struggling with the awful syndrome for almost twenty years, I managed to control it by going on a strict sugar-free and yeast-free diet and a three-month protocol of Diflucan, an antifungal drug. To treat my nerve pain, I had tried medications like Elavil, Lyrica, Neurontin, and Prozac but saw no significant relief; instead, I suffered the cognitive side effects like confusion, fatigue, and a feeling of being detached from my body. Chronic pain is draining, and I knew I couldn't endure being in pain while feeling foggy or tired. After all, my above-average energy level was often what helped me cope with the pain.

In moments like these, when everything seemed too difficult, I was thankful for my mother's medical knowledge, the inner strength she had passed onto me, and her reassuring way. Mom helped me to feel safe and to deal with the uncertainty and risks I often faced due to my connective tissue disease and fibromyalgia. Tom and Audrey were also just a phone call away.

Plus, I now had Bunny Boy. He was a godsend. His companionship, lighthearted persona, and own medical issues kept me from dwelling on mine. Nevertheless, on the day I received the phone call, I just wanted to feel sorry for myself. Our vacation to Kiawah Island, South Carolina, which we had planned in November during New Jersey's school closures for the annual teacher's convention, was rapidly approaching, and I didn't want to cancel. I felt like I was in the middle of a bad rerun. We were going away, no matter what.

I lit the gas fireplace in the living room, grabbed the pale-green chenille blanket off the sofa, and propped myself up, prepared for a good cry. But Bunny Boy came binkying through the archway and across the rug, ruining my plan. I had to smile. Though he was clearly in pain after his surgery, Bunny Boy was still playful and affectionate, and he certainly didn't mope. The penicillin shots and diarrhea seemed like nothing out of the ordinary for our rabbit—just a blip on the radar screen. So, I took Bunny Boy's approach.

"It's just a little inflammation," I told myself, reaching down to pick him up. Yet, this time it seemed more serious than it had been in the past. I was finding it difficult to sit up for any length of time, let alone stand up on my own, and the softest pillow against my back felt like sandpaper, irritating my nerve endings.

Dr. Pasik, whom I had come to regard as my life saver after I was referred to her when I suffered from acute parvovirus years back, doubled my dose of the steroid prednisone, and prescribed for me Voltaren, a different class of anti-inflammatories. I worried about adding Voltaren, which was notoriously hard on the gastrointestinal tract and could cause gastric bleeding. But what choice did I have? Celebrex, another anti-inflammatory we had tried, had been temporarily pulled off the market as new information emerged that there was a correlation between its use and heart attacks. With heart disease running in my family, I was glad to be off of that. We also tried a new pain cream compounded by our local pharmacy and consisting of Tramadol, Lidocaine, Neurontin, and Baclofen. And, of course, many hot packs came out of our medicine drawer.

Tina took on a few more responsibilities around the house, god bless her, and Mom made dinners for us and spent even more time with the kids, taking them to their various afterschool activities. I rested as much as possible while holding Bunny Boy captive, forcing him to listen to audiobook excerpts from *Watership Down* for the tenth time. The exquisite descriptions of the wild rabbits' adventures were intoxicating. He had to enjoy them as much as I did.

A week into my accelerated treatment program, it happened—a day I would never forget. It was Monday morning. Ward had left for work and the children were at school. Tina had taken the day off and wouldn't return until Tuesday morning. After an unusually long and difficult night of intense body pain and sweating, I lay in bed with the phone nearby so I could reach out to a few friends to keep from losing my mind. Bunny Boy was nestled on my chest, content as a little snuggle bug.

When I finally needed to go to the bathroom, I tried to lift Bunny Boy off to get up—but I couldn't move. It felt like I was paralyzed. There was a disconnect between my brain and my body, and I was trapped inside. A sense of sheer panic hit me, an adrenaline rush, and I could feel my eyes widen as if I had just seen something shocking. I was terrified. What if there was a fire and I couldn't get out of bed?

One of the first things that went through my mind was that I was temporarily paralyzed from Guillain-Barré, a virus my doctors periodically checked me for. I had seen Guillain-Barré strike a friend a few years back, paralyzing her for days. I pushed away the unimaginable possibility and tried to reach for the phone. My arms and legs felt as though they were tied to cement blocks, but I was able to move the slightest bit.

"Bunny Boy, I need the phone," I cried out desperately, a little incredulous at my words. I knew a dog might understand what I was saying, but even though Bunny Boy was highly intelligent, I wasn't sure he would.

"Bunny Boy, Mommy needs the phone," I repeated anxiously, praying that someone was watching over me. "Let's play," I added with great foresight, encouraging him to play with the phone and hoping he would inadvertently knock it in my direction.

Bunny Boy popped onto all fours and leaned back on his haunches. We locked eyes. He stared down at my sweaty face. His eyes spoke to me. I believe he sensed something was wrong. Patches of his fur were moist and matted down from my sweat. He started sniffing my face almost in fast motion, like a dog might. It seemed he was trying to figure out what was going on and what to do.

"Buddy, please, get me the phone."

By some miracle or amazing coincidence, Bunny Boy reached his front paws down and turned his head toward me, keeping the rest of his body flush against my stomach as if to reassure me that he wasn't going anywhere, while he nudged the phone closer toward my hand. Tears rushed down my cheeks as I watched this beautiful animal bring me the help I needed. I tried to lift the phone, successfully, but it felt as heavy as a brick. I was blubbering amidst my terror, telling Bunny Boy how much I needed him and how grateful I was.

You're able to move now, so just stay calm, I tried to convince myself. *There's no need to call an ambulance. It can't be that bad.* But my fear was bigger than me. My father would have never survived his first heart attack had the ambulance not gotten to our home in time.

I dialed two of my neighbors, hoping to get another human being in the house as quickly as possible. Nobody answered. How I ached for my mother or sister, but Mom was in Colorado visiting Tom and Carol was at work. I successfully called a dear close friend, Lisa, who lived about ten minutes away. Then I called Ward. Finally, they were on their way over. I dropped my arm that held the phone to the side out of sheer exhaustion and began to pray. *Dear God, I need your help.*

Within minutes, Lisa had used the garage code to let herself into the house. When she came into the room, Bunny Boy was lying in the crook of my neck, sensing, the way a steadfast companion might, that he needed to stay close to me. Every few minutes, he would reach his head up to nuzzle my cheek, letting me know I wasn't alone.

"I am so weak I can barely move, Lisa!" I sobbed. "Nothing like this has ever happened before."

"I am here, Nance," she said in that cheerful voice I had come to rely on to keep me positive during difficult times. There was nothing I couldn't share with Lisa.

"I need to go to the bathroom, but there's no way I can get there. I don't have the strength." I couldn't believe the words that were coming out of my mouth. This was not Nancy. I was stronger than this.

Without a moment's hesitation, Lisa lifted me up tenderly and carried all one hundred and twenty pounds of dead weight to the bathroom.

"I knew you were sick, Nance, but I'm not sure I really understood just how sick," she whispered, gently pushing a sweaty strand of hair off my face. My body started to shake and the beads of perspiration dripped down from my forehead.

With no rush-hour traffic, Ward made it home quickly. He ran into the bedroom with a mixture of fright and sadness on his face. I had never called him at work and said the words "You need to come home" before—except for the time Chris fell off the swings and needed stitches while my car was in the shop.

We drove to the rheumatologist. I lay in the backseat of the car. By that point, I was able to sit up, but I wanted to conserve my physical energy. I walked into the reception area at a turtle's pace, Ward by my side, feeling as though I had run fifty miles with a full load of camping gear on my back.

"We need to talk seriously about starting methotrexate," said Dr. Pasik in her calm, low-pitched voice, which I had grown to appreciate. Methotrexate was a form of chemotherapy. In the past five years, it had showed great promise treating some autoimmune diseases by suppressing chronic inflammation in the body. At the correct dose and proper monitoring, it was effective and reasonably safe. I had done extensive research on it myself, knowing that, at some point, I would probably have to go on it. But I had hoped to avoid it until it was absolutely necessary. Both of the medicines we discussed can be toxic to your liver, kidneys, and blood, and they alter the proper functioning of the very complicated immune system. In my weakened state, part of me wanted to start one of the medications right away, but the logical part was still fearful and not quite ready to make the leap.

"Let's give you an injection of steroids and up your oral dose and see how you feel in a few days. If you are not feeling dramatically better, we will start the methotrexate, but in the meantime let's get some comprehensive blood work."

I knew that, along with the usual blood work, she had to make sure I didn't have tuberculosis. We had a plan.

Miraculously, the prednisone did its job. Within a few days, I was feeling somewhat stronger, and by late October I was markedly better. My pain had decreased, even though I had not regained all of my energy.

"We're going," I announced emphatically, feeling well enough to continue with our vacation plans to Kiawah Island.

Ward suggested that we invite our babysitter, Kelsey, to help out with the kids. Bunny Boy would be staying at my mother's house for the first time. My mom's dog and cat had recently both died within two months of each other, and she and Carol were begging for Bunny Boy's company.

And so we planned for a smooth, restful week. But we neglected to factor in that our tall, beautiful babysitter, with her flowing sandy-brown hair, striking brown eyes, and knock-'em-dead legs, would be a boy magnet. Kelsey started out the trip as an extra set of hands—and ended up being an extra set of problems. Like any normal seventeen-year-old, she wanted to spend most of her time with the teens at the pool or the beach and not with our run-of-the-mill family of four. Throughout the vacation, Kelsey and her rented bike would be missing for extended periods of time, leading up to an alarming night of frantic phone calls, a discovery of missing alcohol from our stash, and finally a knock on our door at one o'clock in the morning where we found her flanked by two resort police officers.

By the time we returned home from the Deep South, having learned how to "shag" and shuck oysters the proper way and cohabitate with palmetto bugs the size of silver dollars, my mother and sister refused to return Bunny Boy.

"He was such wonderful company and barely any work," my mom marveled. Throughout our vacation, I had, of course, called my mother several times to check on him, and my cell phone was filled with pictures of Bunny Boy enjoying his new playground. I was not sure who looked happier, him or my mother.

"Can we keep him one more day?" she begged.

"Please bring him back tonight. Julie and Chris are anxiously awaiting his return."

"Just Julie and Chris?" she teased.

My mother came over toting a sack of new toys for Bunny Boy. At home, our lagomorph was welcomed and greeted with more pomp and circumstance than the president. We had all missed him.

"Bunny Boy is so special," Mom said with a glimmer in her eyes that told me she yearned for another pet of her own. "Some animals come to us for a reason."

"I believe he did," I replied. "Bunny Boy and I were meant to find each other. I cannot remember life without him."

I tucked him close to my chest and told him how much I missed him and how happy he made me. Sweetly, Bunny Boy nudged my chin with his twittering nose and rested his head on my shoulder, like a toddler glad to see its mommy.

"He'll continue to keep an eye on you, honey, much like Flop did with your father," Mom said.

"He already does," said Ward without a moment's hesitation.

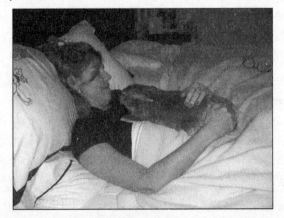

Chapter 13

Soon, the holidays were upon us. Fall was my second favorite time of the year, after Christmas, for decorating and homemaking. A fire burned in our hearth and the smell of embers and a pumpkin candle permeated the air. Bunny Boy's fur was actually a combination of beautiful autumnal shades, and I found the warm colors soothing. Fall was also a time for cooking hearty meals, and just about every meal in our house had something made from pumpkin or apples!

By the time Thanksgiving came each year, we were all tired of eating pumpkin muffins, apple pancakes, and other assorted seasonal items. This year's holiday was no different. We hung out in the family room, still feeling the effects of the tryptophan from our Thanksgiving turkey the day before, relieved that the last pumpkin had been tossed in the garbage. In keeping with tradition, I had prepared our usual Thanksgiving feast for my small extended family of twenty. Ironically, it seemed like less work with the added fun of watching Bunny Boy knock things out of cabinets as I reached for the mixer or as he slid around in bits of flour or sugar that I spilled! Like most years, we had much to be grateful for, and Bunny Boy was the focus of our gratitude this year.

I looked up from my magazine. Ward was relaxed on the sofa while Julie and Chris huddled over the computer playing "Where in the World is Carmen Sandiego?" I felt a peacefulness and closeness with my family. Daily life was often hectic, and I relished our quiet time together. Bunny Boy was stretched out on top of the air duct next to the fireplace, his whiskers fluttering rapidly from the heat. Ward flashed me a playful look of envy when he saw my facial expression of pure adoration for Bunny Boy.

"Why don't we take some pictures of Bunny Boy with the children for the annual Christmas card?" he said.

Even the kids looked up in surprise. Our annual Christmas card was a controversial issue every year. I always wanted a family photo, but no one else did. I had already planned to bring up the topic in early December, hoping that, with a bunny on board, I would get greater cooperation. But Ward had beat me to it.

Ward enthusiastically pulled out his new digital camera from the drawer, a gift from a client. For a moment, I wondered if the spirit of my father had entered Ward's body. My dad loved sending and receiving Christmas cards, as well as bringing in the mail during the Christmas season. When Flop was alive, we would hear him tell her how many cards he thought were in the pile. Every year, the Buchalski family pitched in to write and send out a hundred Christmas cards while sipping hot chocolate and eating Twinkies or Ring Dings as the yule log burned on the television set. Ward, on the other hand, had not grown up with the tradition of Christmas cards, and he hated the bickering that took place in our household when Julie and Chris were old enough to voice an opinion on the matter.

"We don't like 'being on display,' or dressed in matching Christmas outfits for all our relatives and friends to see," they would complain.

But this time was different. There was a unanimous burst of excitement and genuine interest. Chris whisked up Bunny Boy and brushed his fur—which had been blown in a million directions by the air vent. Julie raced up to her room and returned wearing a different shirt and light-pink lip gloss. Her light-brown hair cascaded down her back instead of being held up in her usual ponytail, which made her look naturally beautiful. I gave up on the notion of waiting to have a Christmas tree in the background, welcoming our positive, spontaneous family spirit instead.

With our new digital camera, we could take as many pictures as we wanted without worrying about the cost of developing the film. Bunny Boy and the kids had a ball arranging themselves in various poses. When it came time to choose from the forty or so pictures, we inspected each

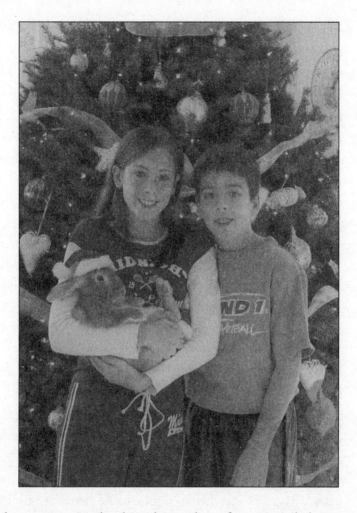

photo like we were Scotland Yard, searching for a pivotal clue in a murder case. Faces lit up, eyebrows furrowed, and jaws dropped!

"We like this one," Ward and Chris cried simultaneously. Out of all of the photos, they had zeroed in on a picture of Julie and Chris holding Bunny Boy in front of the living room fireplace. The lighting was perfect. The setting was lovely.

"But it's X-rated!" I said, half joking. Julie had her arms around Bunny Boy's torso while his thumper legs hung low, exposing his jewels. "No way!"

"Watch this!" said Ward, winking at the kids. He popped the chip back into the camera, tweaked a few buttons, and in a matter of seconds,

Bunny Boy was electronically neutered and patches of soft white fur covered his splendid male anatomy. Technology was amazing.

In keeping with our theme, we enjoyed a very "bunny" Christmas, too. Our lagomorph had his own red velvet stocking with white fur trim on the fireplace next to ours, full of edible seasonal treats. Julie and Chris had picked out everything. It warmed my soul watching them experience a different kind of love—the love for a pet. I had bought a few rabbit ornaments for the Christmas tree and a bunny doorknocker. Bunny Boy wasn't sure what to make of our two Christmas trees. He gazed at the twinkling lights from afar, hesitating to investigate them further. I worried he might chew the needles or tug at the lights and ornaments, but my fears—at least for this first year—were unfounded. For my Christmas gifts, Julie bought me a black T-shirt with a picture of a bunny dragging a Christmas tree by his teeth, and Chris bought me a package of bunny socks with six different neon color combinations.

• • •

Throughout fall and winter, we had also been enjoying the children's sports season. Because I grew with an athletic mother and a father who coached my brothers' Little League teams, sports had always been an important part of my life. As a young girl, I joined Memorial Cadets, the town color guard—first as a flag girl and then as a proud rifle twirler. I quit track tryouts the second week when I jumped over our boxwood hedges from the grass to the driveway practicing hurdles, instead of the reverse, breaking my two front teeth on the concrete. In high school, I wanted to try something new. I joined the dance club and cheerleading. I also made the gymnastics team. Though I had never had formal gymnastics training, I was naturally flexible and eager to put my backyard tumbling to work. And, with the prodding of my five-foot-short, one-hundred-pound mother who played field hockey and basketball in the late 1940s, by junior year I had overcome my fear of the bigger athletic girls and played field hockey for one season. Looking back, I wonder how my parents found the time, let alone the discretionary income, to always support us children in our endeavors.

And now at this point in our family's life, Ward and I were experiencing similar pleasure and fulfillment through our children. Sitting at Chris's soccer games on crisp, sunny days so typical of fall brought me great joy, as did watching Julie progress at her gymnastics and dance lessons. And seeing Bunny Boy learn new tasks like climbing the stepstool or prying open the cabinet door where I kept his corn sticks and other snacks was the icing on the cake!

Basketball season that year was a special one for the Laracy family. Letters had been sent out from the Franklin Lakes recreation center—they were in desperate need of coaches for the grammar school boys' teams. With Chris's help, I set a plan into motion one night, and poor Ward walked through the door right onto a land mine.

"Hey, Dad, Johnny's father says he'll coach our basketball team this year if you'll be his assistant." He gave Ward a hearty slap on the back. "What do you think?"

"Is that right?" Ward replied nonchalantly, opening some of the mail he had brought in. Jonathan was Chris's best friend, and his father, Dan, was an attorney who had the same demanding work schedule as Ward. Neither man had ever played an organized team sport and yet were to coach the boys' teams.

As we sat down for dinner, the phone rang. As part of our brilliant plan, I let Ward answer it. Jonathan had been instructed to tell his father that Ward was interested in coaching this year and was hoping Dan would be his assistant coach. No more than a minute into their conversation, Ward looked right at me.

"Well, Dan, I think we've just been set up. Chris told me that *you* were coaching the boys, not me, and that you were looking for an assistant. I smell a rat, my friend."

Chris kicked me under the table. "Bunny Boy can be the team mascot," I whispered to him. The idea had just come to me.

"If we coach together, we'll make sure we have the boys on the same team, Dan," Ward said, with resignation. But the excitement I sensed in his voice told me that he was ready to be Chris's coach, regardless of how difficult it might be. "With our busy schedules and lack of experience, we can make it work."

While Dan and Ward had a keen interest in watching the NBA basketball games and often made it to the last half of their son's games after work, their coaching credentials were seriously lacking. Most of the dads who coached had been college players themselves and were all trying to relive their youth, it seemed. Dan and Ward just tried to show up on time.

By late January, basketball season was in full swing, and the city lawyers' boys' team, the Mohawks, had a wealth of talent. Dan and Ward had either gotten lucky in the draw or they knew more about basketball than I thought. Or, perhaps it was the luck of our furry mascot, who came to the games.

We had record-breaking snow that winter. Luckily, Bunny Boy loved a good snowstorm. He developed an infatuation with the magical white powder, which made him even more irresistible. He'd lie on his belly with his nose up against the French doors in the sunroom and gaze at the snowflakes as they fell—in awe of their natural beauty. Sometimes, he'd glide his front paws along the glass panes on either side of the front door, as if trying to feel one of the fluffy, white flakes, or he'd popcorn out of sheer excitement, leaving paw prints on the moist glass.

I, too, used to love the snow. When I grew up, the five Buchalski kids spent a lot of time in the woods sledding with very little, if any, parental supervision. On the snow-covered Rainbow Lake in Haskell each year, Carol and I would ice skate with our friends while the boys played hockey. Then, my brother Jack and I would skate together, pretending to be the famous professional ice-skating pair, the Protopopovs. Once I got married, Ward and I took up downhill skiing, which made me love the snow all the more. I felt like I was in heaven when we skied down the bucolic, tree-lined, snow-packed trails in New England or traversed the famous knee-deep powder in the "Back Bowls" at Vail in Colorado.

After I got sick, if my health allowed and I was willing to brave the pain afterward, I would ice skate with Julie and Chris on Lily Pond near our house, twirling and pirouetting across the ice to show off. While I still admire the beauty and elegance of a snowstorm, more moisture and cold means more pain and stiffness. But no matter how cold or inclement the weather was, I went to every one of Chris's winter basketball games. And I was grateful to have the comfort of Bunny Boy's soft, warm body on my lap, which helped lessen my pain as I sat on the hard bleachers cheering on my son. On the nights that Dan and Ward were running late, Bunny Boy would sit in his basket on the stands while I supervised drills for the boys until the real coaches showed up.

The Mohawks were stacking up wins left and right by the end of February, keeping things interesting. On the night of one of Chris's important games, I prepped an Italian dinner for the family. The kitchen table was covered in a classic red-and-white tablecloth, and matching napkins were secured in the middle by red napkin rings I had made by wrapping thick, silk ribbon around plastic shower curtain rings. My pot of Sunday sauce and meatballs was simmering on the stove, creating a delicious aroma in the air.

"Mom, are you cooking for the whole neighborhood?" Chris asked, throwing and catching a basketball on its way up and lunging forward, as if he were about to pass the ball to one of his teammates down the line.

I looked down. My giant pot of meatballs was enough to feed a small village.

"Dinner will be ready at five thirty," I announced. It was four o'clock. "Chris has a seven o'clock game."

I organized my ridiculous amount of meatballs and sauce into eight plastic containers, leaving enough for us simmering on the stove. But when I opened the freezer, I realized there wasn't enough room for all the containers, so I called my neighbor, Nancy, to see if she had any space in her freezer, promising her one container in return for storage rights.

Quickly, I threw on my white ski jacket and stacked three containers of meatballs in my arms like a tower. I opened the door and looked out into the darkness of the evening as the bitter cold air hit my face. *Hmm,* I thought. *Do I walk around the shoveled sidewalk to the side street and cross the road in front of our house—the long way—or do I trudge through the deep snow on the front lawn, cutting my time and distance in half?*

I took the shortcut, trying to use the carved-out footsteps from the UPS man as my path, hearing the frozen snow crunching beneath my feet. Then, as I tried to balance my tower of meatballs, I missed the center of his steps and slipped where the curb met the street. I plummeted onto the asphalt, landing face down on top of the containers. My knees slammed into the ground first, then my shoulder, and finally my head. It was a miracle I didn't break my teeth. The weight of my body crushed the containers open—I found myself lying in meatballs and sauce.

I wanted to scream. I pried myself halfway up, balancing on my knees with the palms of my hands on the asphalt. I tried to wipe the sauce from my face so I could see, but my sauce-covered hands made things worse. Sauce was dripping from everywhere and crystallizing in the nine-degree weather. My pants had ripped and I could feel my knee bleeding. There was barely a sliver of a moon and very few streetlights, and I could hardly see. I tried to gain my composure, but I was angry and cold. My head was throbbing, and quickly, things other than my head began to hurt.

I looked toward the house. Bunny Boy was sitting upright in our dimly lit foyer, waiting for me to come back. His cute little face peeking through the glass was the only thing that kept me from freaking out.

Shaking excess sauce off my clothes and kicking the containers aside with disgust, I limped across the lawn and rang the bell to be let back in as our front door automatically locked behind you. Chris swung the door open. "Julie, hurry, Mom's bleeding!"

"It's not blood! It's tomato sauce!" I said, though it was actually both.

I stumbled into the foyer, almost tripping over Bunny Boy. Now I could see that my fake UGG boots were a psychedelic mess and my white ski jacket was covered in sauce and gravel. Bunny Boy was already lapping up the sauce as it dripped onto the floor. Chris covered his mouth, trying, unsuccessfully, not to laugh. By the time Julie came down, Bunny Boy was sloshing back and forth in a red puddle, which had formed near my ankles on the hardwood floors. He rolled over onto his back and bounced up onto all fours, completely covered. Tomato sauce dripped from his tall ears, whiskers, and nose. He started sneezing, splattering the sauce everywhere. The foyer looked like a war zone.

Bunny Boy tried to wipe his nose and head with his front paws in that adorable way that bunnies do, and it was just the right amount of cuteness I needed. I broke out laughing at the absurdity of it all. His fluffy cottontail was bright red and dragging on the floor from the weight of sauce. His ginger-colored fur was scarlet.

"Go eat your dinner and get into your basketball clothes, Chris. Julie, can you please clean up Bunny Boy?"

She looked at me as if to say, "How?"

I limped up the stairs, took some Advil from the medicine cabinet, and tried to assess my injuries. There was nothing catastrophic; I had suffered worse. I showered and came downstairs, clothed and bandaged. Chris was waiting for me in his basketball uniform, holding two containers of meatballs he had rescued and a large spoon.

The phone rang a minute later. It was Nancy, wondering where her dinner was. "Look out your window," I said. "It's in the street."

While the team mascot stayed home and received a full spa treatment, Chris and I made it to his game by the end of the first quarter. The Mohawks ended up winning first place in the intermediate basketball league. Jonathan and Chris both won MVP, and Bunny Boy won Most Valuable Pet.

"We should give up coaching now," said Ward, handing Dan the trophy. "Anything else is going to be a letdown."

Chapter 14

We were quickly becoming known in town as the Bunny Family. And I was the leader of the pack. Once, I snuck Bunny Boy into Home Depot on a shopping trip, despite a "No pets allowed" sign. We were "caught" by a security guard, who, when he realized Bunny Boy was not a dog, said, "How ya doin', little fella?" and proceeded to help me find my supplies. Once noticed by the rest of the store, Bunny Boy basked in the attention of a dozen (female) customers, clearly enjoying the limelight, and edged onto my shoulder, practically waving goodbye to his fans. Another time, I snuck him into a McDonald's where I was meeting my mother for lunch, where he relished, again, the attention of a couple of octogenarian strangers.

Bunny Boy had quickly become a point of interest and a near celebrity in our community. One day, my neighbor Karen came over to enlist my advice. "Oh come on!" she exclaimed, when I greeted her at the door. "Every time I see you, Bunny Boy is in your arms." It was true. I had been known to answer the door with his head on my shoulder like I was burping a baby. His soft body was food for my soul.

Karen had just bought a bunny for Easter and was hoping to pick my brain on how we had trained an indoor bunny. My first playful thought was, *copycat!* I thought back to Jaws, her vicious outdoor bunny, who, I assumed, had since crossed the rainbow bridge into pet heaven. I sat down to chat with her, enjoying her witty conversation and laughing so hard I could barely keep up with her punchlines. Karen was one of the funniest people I had ever met, and her new bunny would give her all new material. She claimed her new bunny had already reduced her wicker furniture on her indoor porch to matchsticks with her overzealous chewing, and I couldn't resist showing off Bunny Boy, who happily demonstrated his obedience and intelligence—not to mention his cuteness—as he lay in my arms and then binkied around the house.

"Oh come on!" Karen said, staring at Bunny Boy in awe. "I want a rabbit like Bunny Boy."

Certainly, Bunny Boy was different.

Julie and Chris, too, enjoyed enlisting Bunny Boy for their own projects. Using the PVC pipes I had bought from Home Depot, Chris meticulously constructed an elaborate bunny maze in the family room. Bunny Boy sniffed the pipes more than once, checking out his new environment, and then he stuck his head in cautiously. When he dodged inside the pipe, he slipped on the plastic surface and scratched the plastic wildly, trying to get his footing while the pipe bobbed from side to side. For a split second, Bunny Boy was sent rolling upside down with his four paws spread-eagled against the roof of the pipe. It was hysterical watching him figure it out! Bunny Boy quickly realized that if he stayed still the pipe would stop bobbing, so he steadied himself and looked in both directions, seemingly calculating which was the shortest way out. Then he pranced out with major bunny attitude like a show rabbit instead of a frightened bunny who had just been rattled and turned upside down. He was a real clown.

Meanwhile, Julie's middle school science fair was coming up—a first for the Laracy family. Our competitive personalities took hold and ideas for Julie's project flowed freely one night at dinner, while Julie remained strangely quiet, pretending to be considering all of our suggestions. Finally, she blurted out, "Bunny Boy is going to be my project."

She had been planning her project secretly for weeks, getting the required permission from her teachers to use a live animal for her exhibit. Our Bunny Boy would be on display in the auditorium at Franklin Avenue Middle School for all to see and meet! Julie was partnering with a classmate, Chloe, who had two outdoor rabbits, Slate and Spitfire. They, however, would not be joining Bunny Boy at the fair due to their fear of strangers, a result of their living outside in a hutch.

The excitement over Julie's project began to build. I often found Julie and Bunny Boy together in her bedroom, the papers for her project scattered on her bed, as she sang a reggae tune to Bunny Boy, "Whatcha gonna do when they come for you?" It was one of her two favorite ways of communicating with him. The other was when she would hold him up under his armpits, looking at him face to face while delivering her usual line, "You're cute. You're fat. You're really dumb, but I love you," before giving him a big smooch on his fat cheeks.

For weeks leading up to the big event, Julie and Chloe spent hours together either in the library doing research or at home combing the Internet for information on lagomorphs—and the red satin species in particular. They compiled and compared notes on the different living arrangements and social lives of their bunnies and designed a poster detailing how and why those living arrangements may or may not have affected their rabbit's health and personality. Slate and Spitfire cohabitated in a wooden hutch all year round, outside in the elements and among predators, and they had limited human contact. Because of that, their natural instincts to be fearful and skittish remained intact. They were known to charge when approached by anyone other than their owners. Thankfully, Slate and Spitfire had each other to snuggle and socialize with. But now that I'd learned firsthand how wonderful and social a rabbit could be living indoors among a human family, I felt terrible when I saw bunnies kept outside in hutches.

While the girls were busy with their project, I did a little—or rather, more than a little—research of my own. The staff at my local Barnes & Noble came to know me by name and learned to prepare my coffee the way I liked it. They welcomed Bunny Boy, too, who usually sprawled out on my lap or on one of their sofas while I read. They never asked if he was a therapy animal. Bunny Boy and I also frequented our town library, flipping through books and striking up conversations with the staff. I threw our pet store bunny guide into the trash and bought a bunny encyclopedia. Then, I studied how to groom, train, and socialize rabbits the right way—not by trial and error, as we had done with Bunny Boy.

I spent a great deal of time focusing on medical ailments that plagued the lagomorph species and found out more than I cared to know. Upper respiratory infections referred to as "snuffles," gastrointestinal problems, teeth issues, and abscesses caused by the bacteria Pasteurella were common among rabbits. Bunny Boy, a chip off the old block, was racking up one health issue at a time.

Julie and I memorized. We organized. I picked Loretta's brain for practical bunny knowledge and discussed real-life bunny emergencies with Dr. Welch. Through our research, we gained a more in-depth understanding of Bunny Boy's body language and his habits—why he thumped, and why he plumped. We learned what color his urine would turn if he ate certain greens—critical information! We skipped over their warnings about loud noises frightening rabbits, which clearly didn't apply to Bunny Boy. Amazingly, he loved the sound of the vacuum, the staccato beeps and noises of video games, and the theme of his favorite television shows (i.e., our favorite shows). He was also intrigued, rather than terrified, by a good thunderstorm.

We also learned why bunnies multiply so fast. Does, famous for their fecundity, spontaneously ovulate during coitus. They become sexually mature after three months and typically give birth to five or six kits with each litter. We also discovered that bunnies over the ripe age of five are considered geriatric and that the smaller breeds of bunnies can live longer than the larger species, much like dogs. Of course, we already knew that the red satin species had a life expectancy of seven to eight years, and that their trademarks were their beautiful satin fur and high level of intelligence.

The morning of the fair, I brought Bunny Boy to Scuffy's to have his nails clipped. It took great restraint on my part not to purchase a pet sweater with an American flag emblem for him to wear—to ensure first prize for the girls! When Julie came home from school, we brushed Bunny Boy's fur and checked his hindquarters for any residual grapelike clusters, then opened his mouth to make sure there were none stuck on his front teeth. Ward raced through the door from work around six, practically inhaled his dinner, and then tested Julie on her facts, trying to trip her up.

The crowds came out in masses that night. I had also invited my siblings and their families—I could always count on their support. It was almost embarrassing. At any given point in time, there was at least one sibling, their spouse, a cousin, or a friend roaming the aisles and saying things to other guests like, "Did you see that gorgeous bunny? He's so domestic and calm. Isn't he terrific?" I had to tell them to stop.

The girls' exhibit was standing room only. Despite all the noise and commotion, our lagomorph sat, relaxed, in Julie's arms while she handed out fact sheets to spectators or strands of hay to him. Chloe handled the verbal presentations, and they both took turns answering questions. I tried discreetly to snap photos of Julie, Chloe, and Bunny Boy from virtually every angle, without success. Chris caught me.

"Take a few more, Mom. We don't have enough." Chris never failed to remind me that we already had almost as many photos of Bunny Boy as our firstborn, Julie. The number of pictures that we had of Chris came in at a distant third.

While the girls didn't win one of the top prizes, they had received the most spectators by a large margin.

I should have bought the sweater.

As I drove home from the fair, it suddenly occurred to me. Had all of the constant commotion in the house caused Bunny Boy to feel stressed, possibly suppressing his immune system; or was he born that way? From the night he came into our life, Bunny Boy had always been in the thick of things. How many times had I heard the phrase "Stress compromises your immune system" directed to myself? Should I have done things differently for him?

Chapter 15

When it was springtime again, I found a nest of baby bunnies in our flowerbed. I would walk past the kits several times a day to check on them, compelled to guard them from predators. Seeing the baby bunnies in their nests reminded me that rabbits are the symbol of rebirth. Spring, itself, is the rebirth of many things. Nature's wonders replace the barrenness of winter. Green leaves burst from buds to engulf the deciduous trees, and perennial flowers sense when it's time to color the landscape. And the wonder of hearing the birds chirp or the owls hoot might cause someone to pause and think, *Is there some higher power?*

The tiny creatures with so little fur and their eyes closed also made me realize how much Bunny Boy had grown. He had lost his yummy baby look—his ginger fur now looked like it had been sprinkled lightly with brown sugar, and the white area around his nose was receding. He maintained his peak weight of eight and a half pounds with a healthy diet made up of mostly timothy hay and a small amount of pellets or fresh greens. Tiny pieces of apples and bananas were reserved for snacks, which he was crazy about. He'd thump if he didn't get his fruit roughly the same time every morning, letting me know he was impatient.

Bunny Boy had reached new heights of lusciousness. I would come home and find him plumped like a hen under the wingback chair next to the fireplace. With the sun on his back, his fur glistened like crystals and his eyes shone like black onyx. Other times, he would be lying on his side, sleeping peacefully under a dining room chair. I would resist the urge to scoop him up and give him a big ole raspberry on his pudgy belly and instead give him a gentle kiss and let him rest. During dusk and early morning when he was most active, he would gambol across the house with sheer delight, eventually landing in my waiting arms!

Bunny Boy's personality continued to emerge, like layers being pulled off an onion. He was extremely gentle, loving, and calm, but also mischievous and independent. He grew more attached to us every day. I found his affection intoxicating, his purring soothing. Bunny Boy would only purr when he was snuggling with Chris or me. But he would only lick me. The first time Bunny Boy licked my hand, Julie insisted it was because he liked my hand cream. Licking is indicative of a deep bond that very few bunnies form with their owners—and the ultimate sign of love from a male bunny is when he sprays you with urine. Then, you become his soul mate.

The love I felt for Bunny Boy was a different type of love, one I had not experienced since my early childhood days with Flop. We would wrestle or cuddle, and I would say the most ridiculous things that felt totally okay: "I love you more than life itself" or "You're the love of my life, Bunny Boy."

Julie was the most bothered by Bunny Boy's affection for me. Ward didn't lose sleep over it, and Chris, with his competitive nature, claimed he and I were neck in neck when it came to vying for Bunny Boy's love. And he was right. My rough and tumbly son had trained Bunny Boy to sleep with him on his bed like I had, a feat Julie had yet to master (her singing kept him awake)! Chris would carry Bunny Boy up to his room and they would wrestle on his bed like true boys until Bunny Boy fell over, as if to say, "I've had enough." Chris would then crawl under his comforter and lie perfectly still, waiting for Bunny Boy to make his move. Like clockwork, Bunny Boy would yank the blanket back with his teeth, just enough to crawl into Chris's armpit as if a magnet was sucking him in. He'd adjust himself every few minutes, tucking his head deeper and deeper into the dark, warm space. It was amazing that he could still breathe, and even more amazing that Chris could stay still for so long.

As the seasons came and went, my children were changing, too. Chris's sandy-brown hair had grown long below his chin, and his physique was toned and muscular. He was chalking up athletic awards as quickly as Bunny Boy was stacking up nicknames—Bunnykins, Bachagaloops, Little Man, Buchykins, or Fluffball. Chris's drive and motivation had served him well in all of his sports, including his newest endeavor, lacrosse. He had just completed his first season and survived with all his limbs intact and a full set of teeth—barely. Chris had also broken the school record back in the fall at the Turkey Trot, the grammar school annual track and field event, finishing the mile run in less than six minutes. My precision-timed "Speedy Gonzales" drills—designed to use up some of his excess toddler energy—had had him racing around the trees in the yard when he was only three years old. They had clearly paid off. For his win, he earned himself a plaque in the entrance hall display cabinet and the ultimate prize, a milk chocolate turkey. One year, helicopter parents fought desperately to cancel the thirty-year tradition, claiming the competition damaged the self-esteem of the slower children and adding that the chocolate turkey was bad for the winner's health. "Why not an apple?" one parent suggested. What child will run fast for an apple? Thankfully, their best efforts failed. Whenever Chris won, I gave him a Russell Stover chocolate rabbit, of course—to go with the turkey!

Meanwhile, at fourteen years old, Julie was beginning to develop curves and softness about her body. Her natural blonde highlights had vanished and her eyebrows were dark and full, set above her deep blue eyes. I was waiting to hear the question, "Can I put purple streaks in my hair?" Julie and her friends were hanging out at Dunkin' Donuts or the mall and less at our house. I missed the girl talk and their clothing swaps, the empty juice boxes and straws strewn on the deck around the hot tub, or their towels slung on the floor by the washing machine. Bunny Boy, no doubt, missed rummaging through the girls' backpacks and purses and scoping out the talent. He'd sit upright on his haunches and watch the girls parade by in their swimsuits as they headed for the outdoor Jacuzzi. Male hormones transcend species.

Julie was also studying for her confirmation, the Christian rite of passage. Her best friend, Amanda, was studying for her bat mitzvah, the Jewish rite of passage. They often complained about how much time was needed to "grow up," as they put it. They were busy tweens. When asked by the priest at her pre-confirmation interview why she wanted to do her confirmation, Julie replied, "Because my parents are making me."

I cringed.

When Father Joe asked her what she thought of the Trinity, Julie said, "I don't believe in any of that stuff!" Stuff? I couldn't imagine what would have happened if I had said something like that to our priest when I was a kid! I am not sure whose wrath would have been worse, the priest's or my parents'.

"I believe what you do in this life comes back to you in another," she added, with a forthright attitude.

A rather mature statement, I thought. While I welcomed Julie's independent spirit, I thought she had crossed the line with regard to showing respect. I was still a bit old fashioned and always strived for respect in our children.

"You mean like in Buddhism? You return in another life as a fly?" Father Joe said curtly.

"Or a rabbit?" I chuckled to myself. Father Joe had yet to meet Bunny Boy, but the other priest, Father Mike, had blessed him twice at the Feast of St. Francis, the patron saint of animals.

When it came to religion, Julie didn't appear to have inherited a single gene of mine. I had loved Catholicism from the time I was a young girl. I sat at mass most mornings before school with my white lace chapel cap bobby-pinned to my hair, and I held my prayer book happily. Every year I dreamed of becoming one of the eight girls chosen to wear the pastel chiffon dresses and lead the May Crowning procession on May 15 to celebrate the Blessed Mother. There were two beautiful dresses of each color—peach, yellow, blue, and green.

In fourth grade, that dream came true. I can still picture the wispy, fresh wreath of flowers, which sat over my Shirley Temple curls, curls my mom created with bobby pins and that she brushed lovingly. I remember the softness of the peach chiffon flowing dress that shaped my undeveloped body. I can still smell the bouquet of white roses and pink lilies I held in my small hands. I felt like a princess that day.

I could only hope that my love of religion would radiate in my being and be passed onto Julie. Living in a melting pot where many religions comingled never failed to raise the question: "Is there one true God, or is one religion more accepted than another?" Teen magazines like *CosmoGirl* featured articles preaching atheist and agnostic principles, backed by statistics, which only confused Julie more. While Ward grew up Catholic and went to twelve years of parochial school, he began to have atheist views in his early twenties. But we had agreed to raise the children Catholic until they made their confirmation—and then they could choose their own path. That was our compromise.

Chris, on the other hand, appeared fine with church and catechism for the time being. He also seemed to enjoy praying, which meant the world to me. Once, when he was about five years old, I remember walking into his bedroom one summer night to say goodnight and found him glassy-eyed, sitting on the edge of his bed, staring out the open window. There was a luminescent, waxing moon high up in the black sky. His dark-green pleated shades with gold stars were flapping from the outside breeze.

"What's wrong honey?" I asked tenderly, hugging him close.

"I usually cry when I pray. Don't you, Mom?" he replied, with the innocence of a small child.

I treasure those moments.

• • •

Up until Julie's birth, Ward and I had assumed I would return to work full-time after three months since my career was such an important part of my life. But within weeks of having Julie wrapped in my arms, we agreed with no hesitation that motherhood would become my new career, at least for a while.

Motherhood suited me almost immediately. Perhaps it was my reward for enduring an extremely difficult pregnancy. With Julie, I felt a great sense of achievement for having survived the pregnancy from hell. Besides throwing up for nine months, I developed placenta previa (a ruptured placenta) during my first trimester and was on complete bed rest. During my second trimester I endured fevers of 101 degrees, and strange rashes appeared on my face and extremities, causing me to end up in the hospital. I had contracted cytomegalovirus (CMV), a virus that had everyone very worried.

Ultimately, Julie was born with antibodies to CMV, but thankfully she did not have any of the serious birth defects it can cause, except for a low birth weight of four pounds and thirteen ounces. Back then, I was also told that I might have lupus or a connective tissue disease, but pregnancy hormones often alter the results of blood work, which made the tests inconclusive. The immunologist even thought I could be dangerously allergic to my own hormones—how ridiculous!

It was a scary time. To keep my ob-gyn on his toes until the bitter end, I developed full-blown toxemia, which necessitated a Caesarean birth three weeks before my due date. I was accused of trying to develop at least one complication from each chapter of the six-hundred-page encyclopedia on pregnancy that I had purchased within hours of seeing the pink line on the home pregnancy test (I read it cover to cover—twice). My ob-gyn told me I had single-handedly turned his hair gray. I was pretty sure I would not be featured on the cover of any natural birthing magazine unless the editors wanted to terrify or lose their subscribers!

But my cherub was worth all the discomfort and angst I had had to live through to bring her into the world. I couldn't imagine life without my Juliebear.

My first priority had always been to be the best mother I could be to our children. With Ward's grueling schedule, I knew my career had to be put on the back burner. I also wanted to emulate my own mother, who I truly believed was the kindest mother in the world. Even so, I still held out hope of returning to executive recruiting one day, even though that opportunity faded even faster with my diagnosis at age thirty-seven. And even after sticking tiny needles into my head and extremities, receiving small jolts of electricity, sleeping on a magnetic mattress, choosing a mantra and speaking to Buddha, having my back and neck cracked, or sending vitamins or hydrogen peroxide flowing through my veins (i.e., trying every holistic treatment available), my overall health was still unpredictable.

In between my times volunteering at the children's schools and nursing homes, I was also studying nutrition and alternative treatments for chronic pain using the Internet, the library, and various medical publications, hoping to design a website and start a web column that could reach the chronic pain community. It was an ambitious endeavor, but I needed to have a plan for the future. Meanwhile, Ward's law firm of eighteen years had merged with a much larger law firm, which would bring about more lucrative, interesting opportunities for him.

It was an exciting time for all of us, including Bunny Boy. At almost two and a half years old, he already had his own book of "baby" firsts. Bunny Boy's milestone events were things like: "Used litter pan. Thumped. Drank from a bowl. Purred for the first time. And licks now, but only his mother." His change of gender was noted along with the mix-up over being a dwarf. The most recent entry read: "Hops onto furniture now. Not sure what took him so long!"

The first time Bunny Boy hopped onto my lap, I was sitting on the recliner, reading. He almost floated up. He seemed surprised himself. I threw my arms around him, pinched his cheeks, and squealed, "My god, you're so precious, Bunny Boy."

Julie looked up from the computer with a sweet expression on her face. "That's kind of cute."

"Kinda cute? It's awesome!" Chris exclaimed, annoyed at his sister's apparent lack of excitement. He practically pushed me off the chair, seeking his own chance to experience Bunny Boy's newest feat.

"Good job, Butchykins," I said, patting his backside. "Do it again, pal!"

Bunny Boy popcorned across the room faster than normal as if to say, "Yippee, look at me!" He returned and stopped about a foot away from the recliner, very deliberately eyeing the distance to the chair. Then, with major bunny attitude, he leapt into Chris's lap. It was a defining moment. The recliner, which we quickly named the "King of the Castle" chair, would become his favorite hangout site. The ground was no longer his only turf.

"You give it a try, Jules," encouraged Chris, looking for the same unbridled enthusiasm from his sister.

"Maybe later, Chris," she said. "I'm working on a school paper."

Julie and Chris were very different children; about as different as Bunny Boy and Sunny. Chris was warm and expressive, but he also needed a lot of attention. He was extremely active, even in utero. As a toddler, I called him my little Houdini. He climbed out of his crib, got over the gate, and stood on the highchair tray all before the age of one. Julie, on the other hand, expressed her emotions in a less obvious way, just like her father. A sunny baby and toddler, she spoke early, walked late, and stayed out of mischief. Most of her fine and gross motor skills lagged due to her premature birth, but she had a fiercely independent spirit from an early age, never showing any signs of separation anxiety or attachment issues.

On the first day of nursery school, Julie walked into the small brick building confidently with her Care Bear backpack, never looking back. Within weeks, we were called in for a formal nursery school conference. "She's very precocious and independent. She doesn't follow directions," said her teacher. Chris, on the contrary, clung to my pants every morning for the first three weeks of preschool. And if he wasn't getting stitches from breaking our glass coffee table with his head, then he was diving off the swing set into the sand and splitting his lip or trying to shave his face with Ward's razor. He was a lovable menace that could push me to the brink of utter frustration or make my heart melt with happiness.

No role was more challenging or rewarding than that of a mother. As mothers, we're supposed to be experts on health, child development, family values, and education without any formal training. We are expected to nurture, teach, and, at times, give up our own identities to be the best mother we can be. So, as I watched Bunny Boy hop onto the furniture for the first time, I felt that familiar wonderment when my own children did something new.

In the days and weeks ahead, Bunny Boy enjoyed seeing the world from a whole new perspective. He hopped onto chairs and traversed the backs of the sofas. He slid across coffee tables and scaled the stairs to the second floor, seeking out new places to nap. He would popcorn down the narrow upstairs hallway, bouncing off the walls and sending the toys Chris had left lying around tumbling down the stairs. He raced in and out of the bedrooms like he was participating in a car chase—though it was Tina, me, or the kids chasing him and not a Ferrari! He pillaged clean loads of laundry that Tina or I had left at the foot of our beds and nearly fell into the toilet when he hopped up and stumbled on the seat. Tina got the biggest kick out of Bunny Boy. *"Muy mal conejo!"* she would joke. Very bad bunny. At dusk, our house seemed to come alive as Bunny Boy embarked on his rampage. From the downstairs kitchen, it sounded like an entire warren of bunnies occupied the second floor and not just a single bunny having a good time!

When you least expected, Bunny Boy would appear like a ninja and spring onto your lap, seeking affection. One night, he floated onto the kitchen table while we were playing family poker and started tapping the faces of Julie's cards with his twittering nose, as if he were giving her a "bunny good luck" sign. He would become a regular player in every one of our poker games, until the night he binkied across the table and knocked over Chris's pile of chips, scaring the daylights out of himself. Then, Bunny Boy watched us play poker from my lap.

In every way, he had become part of our family. *How wonderful this bunny was,* I thought, *for me and for all of us.*

Chapter 16

When I saw it, I bolted upright on the sofa. "My god, it's back, Ward!" I shrieked.

"What's back?"

"Bunny Boy's abscess."

The unsightly lump was the size of a golf ball. I was instantly heartbroken. I had hoped that Bunny Boy would never have another abscess. I drew him close and whispered in his long, beautiful ears.

"Everything is going to be okay, Bunny Boy. I promise."

Now, I just had to convince myself,

It was a Sunday night during early fall. *Sixty Minutes* was wrapping up a segment on helicopter parents. Chris and Julie were sitting on the floor organizing a pile of Pokémon cards. When he heard my yell, Chris jumped up and came over to us.

"It's small compared to the last one," he said in a sullen voice. "His other one was the size of a tennis ball."

"Your mother will make sure Bunny Boy gets the best medical care," Ward said, with the conviction that said he had complete faith in me.

I spent the night on the couch in the lagomorph lounge, formerly known as our family room. After all, the largest space in the house had been taken over by Bunny Boy's toys, and the name change seemed appropriate. The cabinets that once housed our family photo albums now stocked bags of hay and litter, while the laundry baskets that were once brimming with Little People buses and fire trucks, My Little Ponies, and Matchbox cars were now full of balls, tunnels, playmats, veggies, and books made out of edible hay.

I needed to be close to Bunny Boy that night. Waiting for Dr. Welch's office to open the next morning seemed like an eternity. We cuddled together in the dark. I put hot compresses on his jaw every few hours, reconciling myself to the fact that Bunny Boy would need another surgery. I would gently palpate the abscess, as if hoping, somehow, that I could make it go away.

Around five in the morning, I woke from a wonderful dream. I had been nestled in a pool of fur—a litter of baby bunnies. When I opened my eyes, Bunny Boy was lying on my chest, purring. His paws and head were tucked under my chin and he stared directly into my eyes with intensity. The warmth of his body felt like heaven, except for the hard lump against my bare neck, which snapped me back to reality.

"You're the love of my life, buddy," I whispered. "I hope you know that."

Bunny Boy lifted his head ever so slowly and twitched his nose against mine like Samantha from *Bewitched*. He started gently licking my cheek as tears began to trickle down. I fell back to sleep, with his soft body against my chest, my face wet with tears.

When I got up around seven o'clock, Bunny Boy was sitting in his litter pan, seemingly content, like the average male taking a dump.

"Good morning, Bunny Boy. How are you feeling, buddy?"

Bunny Boy flew enthusiastically out of his pan and up onto the sofa, landing on my chest on all fours, as if trying to convince me that everything was alright, much like he had when I received the dreadful news about Audrey. He was active and alert, his usual cheerful self. He never skipped a beat.

The morning was less chaotic than usual. Everyone did their part keeping the mood in the house upbeat. Ward made the kids breakfast and prepared their lunches. Chris heated the rolled towel in the microwave and Julie checked it, making sure it wasn't too hot, so I could do another hot compress on Bunny Boy. I called the animal hospital and left a detailed message for Dr. Welch, who was in her Monday morning surgeries. Then I called my siblings. I did a few household chores, with Bunny Boy at my heels, and answered emails with him on my lap. Then I said the rosary.

Dr. Welch returned my call around noontime.

"I'd like you to consider bringing Bunny Boy into the Animal Medical Center in New York City."

New York? Why couldn't she perform the surgery? Dr. Welch must think this recurrence very serious.

"They're using a new cutting-edge treatment for these types of abscesses," she said with an optimism I desperately needed to hear. Dr. Welch had watched the procedure being performed at the University of Pennsylvania, but she did not know how to perform it herself. She continued, "I think Bunny Boy is the perfect candidate for this surgery. The veterinarian will implant granular antibiotic beads into his jawbone once they remove the abscess, and the antibiotic will be absorbed slowly and directly into the area over a period of three months. Combined with adjunct antibiotic therapy, this procedure may dramatically change the course of these stubborn abscesses."

Her last words were all I needed to hear. I hung up the phone, feeling a great sense of hope.

I called the exotic department at the Animal Medical Center (AMC) and took the first available appointment for seven a.m. the next day. No doubt Bunny Boy was one of a kind, but *exotic* was never an adjective we had used to describe him. A new nickname would surely be in his future.

The next morning, Bunny Boy and I slipped out of the house quietly at five fifteen. He sat in the front seat of the car, looking out of the windows into the darkness. His abscess was painfully visible. Donna, another one of my devoted friends, was waiting to be picked up at our local Dunkin' Donuts with two cups of coffee. She had kindly agreed to accompany me. Within minutes, Bunny Boy relaxed in her lap with his chin leaning on the console.

We crossed the George Washington Bridge and headed downtown on Harlem River Drive with time to spare. The AMC was located on First Avenue and 62nd street, twenty-eight blocks north of the New York University office of my second rheumatologist, Dr. Brown, who had become part of my own treatment team over the last year or so. I had gone to NYU for a second opinion after the option of methotrexate, a form of chemotherapy, or a biologic like Enbrel seemed close to becoming a reality, back when I had experienced my episode of near-paralysis.

Bunny Boy and I made a memorable entrance. I slipped in a puddle of pet urine that had yet to be cleaned up and crashed into the reception desk. Bunny Boy dug his paws deep into my chest trying to hang on.

"Bunny Boy Laracy!" I announced.

We took our seats among a group of diverse pet owners and their pets. They don't call New York a melting pot for no reason. There were several large dogs with missing limbs, a cat with very little fur left on her skinny body that exposed the vertebrae on her back, two colorful birds, and a few lapdogs. Nothing exotic, at least until we showed up. Doctors and technicians milled around holding charts, giving post-operative instructions, or simply offering a caring word. It was like being at Columbia Presbyterian or Sloane-Kettering Hospital, but for animals.

To my right sat a woman who could have been a young version of the Queen of England, hat and all.

"She has to be British," I mumbled to myself. A miniature Chihuahua was bulging out of her Louis Vuitton purse.

"Munchkin Wells, please?" inquired one of the physicians, looking around for her pet patient. "Munchkin Wells?"

I nearly burst into laughter. I knew who they were looking for.

"That woman's face could be on the label for an Earl Grey teabag," I said, nudging Donna.

The woman walked toward the doctor with perfect posture and poise, balancing her hat, purse, and Taco Bell–style dog.

"Here we are, ma'am." Her accent was as elegant and beautiful as she was. "Be still, Munchkin," she whispered, shoving the dog down into her pocketbook, which struck me as out of character for a woman with such class. "Let's not be naughty."

After Munchkin left, being the social creature that I am, I turned to make conversation with the male couple on our left and their enchanting little dog, a Pomeranian who was the same color as Bunny Boy.

"It's an ungodly hour to be at the vet," I said, reaching to pet the darling dog. "What's his name?"

"He's a she, and her name is Elizabeth. Mine is Bruce," the man replied. "This is Sal, my life partner. Elizabeth loves having two dads." I was not surprised to find a puppy with two dads here in New York.

"My name is Nancy, and this is Donna." We all shook hands.

"How about your little love? What's the bunny's name?"

"His name is Bunny Boy," I answered.

"Bunny Boy's cuddling like a baby," Sal said, with a glimmer in his eyes.

Instinctively, I pulled Bunny Boy to my chest and covered him with both arms as a Doberman Pinscher and his owner came out of the elevator into the lobby. "His bark is worse than his bite," the gentleman said, yanking the dog's chain but struggling to keep him from ending up on my lap. Elizabeth yapped loudly in the Doberman's face, and he retreated with his tail between his legs. A strong-willed, fearless little female dog. I loved her already.

"Is Elizabeth very sick?" I asked, after a moment's hesitation.

"Oh gosh, no, sweetie. Elizabeth's just here for her well checkup. We bring her twice a year."

A well checkup? I had just assumed that most of the pets were here for serious health issues.

"Please don't tell me your little love is sick?" the couple asked. I pointed to Bunny Boy's jaw. The abscess looked like it had gotten larger.

"Bunny Boy will need aggressive surgery to save his life," I said sadly. "He has an incurable abscess."

"My god, Sal, we need to pray," Bruce shrieked. "We all need to pray." He started waving his hands to get people's attention. "Hello, excuse me, excuse me. May I have everyone's attention, please?" Everyone in the room looked up. "We all need to pray at once for—what did you say his name was?"

"Bunny Boy," I said sheepishly.

"Bunny Boy. We all need to pray for Bunny Boy."

Everyone dropped his or her heads in prayer. It was incredibly touching.

Sal was a hairdresser who designed wigs for children with cancer. Bruce ran a deli. They were a very loving couple, and Elizabeth was obviously spoiled. She wore a sweater with the signature Moschino red heart on the front, and her carrying case had the Chanel logo stamped on the side. Her fur was long and wispy, and she darted back and forth between her dads' laps, spinning and twirling like she had just drunk a bowl of Red Bull instead of water.

"So, where's your girls' apartment?" asked Bruce.

"Our apartment?" I said. Then it dawned on me.

"Nance," Donna whispered, figuring it out at the same time. "They think we're a couple." She quickly offered to the group, "My husband has his office here in the city on 44th and Fifth Avenue."

"I live in New Jersey with my husband, about forty minutes from here," I added.

"My, you've come a long way!" said Bruce, without skipping a beat. "Bunny Boy, you have suuuch a good mommy, don't you?"

"Elizabeth has her own lavender bathroom. Lavender's her favorite color," Sal said, with a seriousness that made me realize he was not kidding. "It's upstairs, off from the spare bedroom."

"How wonderful," I said, thinking about poor Julie who had to share her bathroom with Chris and the dirty clothes and moldy towels he left on the floor. "Lucky Elizabeth."

Sal reached sweetly for his partner's hand. "Does Bunny Boy have his own little bathroom?"

I glanced at Elizabeth—her two dads, her sweater, her carrying case. My competitive spirit emerged. I had to do it.

"The beige bathroom off from the kitchen is his," I lied.

In reality, Bunny Boy hated the beige bathroom. During his first morning in the house, he had slipped on the marble floor and avoided that bathroom ever since.

"He also has a sweater with an American flag on the front," I fibbed in a playful manner. I *should* have bought that sweater after all. Donna rolled her eyes in disbelief. I thought to myself, *My god, what am I saying?* I had succumbed to peer pressure and told two egregious lies.

"Bunny Boy Laracy, please?"

In the nick of time, I was rescued from my deceitful behavior by a technician.

I followed the woman down the corridor into an examination room. My decision not to use a carrier hadn't gone unnoticed.

"Backup in room three! We have a bunny," I heard someone say from the hallway. I felt like I was in the middle of a drug raid.

"I guess we made a memorable entrance, buddy."

The veterinarian walked in a few minutes later, addressing Bunny Boy, not me.

"Hello, Bunny Boy. I'm Dr. Hess."

"Where's Franklin Lakes?" she asked me, reaching to shake my hand. Back before *The Real Housewives of New Jersey* made its debut in the spring of 2009 and tarnished the reputation of the town, the suburban oasis was tucked quietly in Bergen County and hidden on the map.

"In Bergen County, New Jersey, about forty minutes west of the city," I replied, puzzled. I thought it was an odd way to start a conversation with a pet owner.

"I see the abscess. We'll get to that later." Her serious tone rattled me. "There are just a few questions I'd like to ask before we start the exam, Mrs. Laracy." She flipped through the manila folder labeled "Bunny Boy," which contained his records that Dr. Welch had faxed over. The barrage of "just a few" questions began, some of which surprised me.

"What was the ancestry of Bunny Boy's mother?"

"I assume she was a red satin," I replied, instead of saying, "How would I know? She abandoned him." I was hoping to shine some levity on the situation to get both of us to relax.

"His father?"

"I believe he must have been a red satin as well. Bunny Boy is a purebred."

"Was Bunny Boy born in this country or abroad?"

"He's a domestic bunny."

"At what age was Bunny Boy weaned?"

"We bought him during a blizzard from a pet store. He was seven weeks old and weaned by then."

"What percentage of Bunny Boy's diet is hay?"

"A lot, right pal?"

"Fresh greens?"

She hadn't seen our vegetable drawer in the refrigerator. There was a science experiment growing inside.

"Does he ingest his cecotropes?"

"He better," I joked.

"Does Bunny Boy drink tap water or bottled water?"

"We have well water."

"Good enough. Does Bunny Boy live outside in a hutch or inside your house?"

"He has free run of our Georgian colonial."

That got her attention.

"I'm happy to hear that," she said with just a hint of a smile. "Our indoor bunnies do better in all respects. They are less stressed."

She continued. "How often does Bunny Boy have his nails taken care of?"

I thought I would try one more time to get Dr. Hess to lighten up. "More often than me." It worked like a charm.

"Probably more often than me, too," she said. "When was his last well checkup?"

"He's never had one," I said, ashamed.

"How often is Bunny Boy brushed?"

"Often. And he enjoys having his fur blow-dried." She looked at me, not sure what to make of my comment.

"I blow-dry his fur after I bathe him."

"Bathe him?" Her tone and facial expression turned serious again. "Bunnies groom themselves. They don't like water. Or loud noises!"

"We've encountered a few different situations that required a bath. Once, he had severe diarrhea from an antibiotic."

"Rabbits are frail, fretful animals, Mrs. Laracy. Bathing is stressful for a bunny. Their hearts are weak."

"Yes, I am painfully aware of that."

"Has Bunny Boy ever had fleas?"

"Of course he's never had fleas," I snapped, without realizing it.

"There are only a few more questions, Mrs. Laracy. I want to be as thorough as possible," said Dr. Hess, sensing I was insulted by the flea question.

Thorough was an understatement. I had been sick for over eight years and had seen a minimum of a dozen specialists in many different fields of medicine, but I had never been asked such pointed questions regarding my diet, hygiene, or, for that matter, my ancestry.

By the time we were done with the questions, the backup SWAT team had arrived. I was also starting to feel more comfortable with Dr. Hess's formal manner. She was clearly very knowledgeable about bunnies, and Bunny Boy and I were both warming up to her.

I handed Bunny Boy over and asked the two assistants to restrain him gently. "He's very docile and cooperative. Bunny Boy will never charge or bite, and there's no need to worry that he will injure you with his hind legs, I promise. He's a perfect gentleman."

Everyone smiled.

The examination fell into the category of something the president of the United States might receive during his own medical checkup. Bunny Boy's individual nails and teeth were checked closely. His genitalia were groped. His ears were examined—externally for mites or fleas and internally for fluid, an infection, or a ruptured eardrum. Dr. Hess listened to Bunny Boy's heart and lungs twice, and then his stomach.

"He seems to eat well," she said, pushing gently on his belly.

Finally, she inspected the abscess like it was a rare gem and got right to the point.

"I'll need to get a cat scan and take some x-rays of his jaw. We'll use a mild sedative. Bunnies tolerate it well, but there is always a slight risk."

"I would prefer that Bunny Boy not have any sedative," I said. "I can hold him very still for the scans."

"It's not our policy to allow an owner in with their pet. I'm sorry."

"Is it a must that Bunny Boy have the scans? Can they operate without them?"

"They serve as a diagnostic map for the surgeon," she replied. "It's very important. We'll take good care of Bunny Boy, I promise."

Reluctantly, I agreed to the cat scan and X-rays, and we were dismissed. About forty minutes later, Dr. Hess came out to the lobby with Bunny Boy wrapped in a blue fleece blanket. He looked like a sleeping angel. Donna and I were both drinking our second cup of coffee of the day. Elizabeth had already left with a clean bill of health.

"He may be groggy for the rest of the day," she said with more warmth, transferring him to my waiting arms. "The abscess is deeply imbedded in Bunny Boy's jawbone at the root of his bottom molar, Mrs. Laracy. It appears the infection may also be in the bone."

I knew it was serious. Back in one of the exam rooms, she showed me the abscess on the X-ray and asked about his first surgery in detail. She wanted to know how quickly he recovered from the anesthesia and whether or not I had trouble with him chewing his stitches. She wondered how well he tolerated the antibiotics and how long it took for him to eat on his own and resume his normal activity. By this time, I was feeling more comfortable with her and knew Bunny Boy would be in good hands.

"The antibiotic beads are our newest line of defense against these types of abscesses. We are extremely hopeful. Right, Bunny Boy?" said Dr. Hess, looking fondly down at my bundle.

My biggest concern was that the surgery required more anesthesia. I knew Bunny Boy would be fine post-operatively. He seemed to be able to handle pain well and had cooperated with the post-surgery protocol. But there was always a risk with anesthesia.

"We can schedule the surgery for next week, Mrs. Laracy, if that works for you?"

"Yes, that would work fine."

With those words, I had also agreed to allow Bunny Boy to be a pioneer of the antibiotic beads. This would not be any regular surgery.

"Please call me any time, day or night, if you have any questions or problems with Bunny Boy. Here's my cell phone number." And she meant it. Not one of my own doctors had ever given me their cell phone number. I looked at her with admiration. She clearly cared deeply for her pet patients.

At the checkout counter, Donna and I read the bill. It was over a thousand dollars, and the surgery was yet to come.

During dinner that night, we discussed Bunny Boy's upcoming procedure. I explained how the antibiotic beads worked and how they would decrease the likelihood of the abscess returning. I also told Julie and Chris that Bunny Boy would be part of important research, which made them happy and proud. Ward reminded me how well Bunny Boy had recovered from his first operation.

"I had to move to the other bedroom to get some sleep, remember?"

Within hours of returning home from the hospital, Bunny Boy was almost too active for his own good. It seemed he had no trouble coming out of the anesthesia just as he had after his first surgery. I cringed, thinking back to that time and picturing him squeezing under the coffee table with his black-and-blue face and swollen head.

"Let's keep doing the hot compresses every day," said Julie.

"I'll help," Chris chimed in. "Bunny Boy's going to help other animals, right?"

"Yes, he will," said Ward.

But I couldn't cheer up. I left most of the food on my plate. When I went to check on Bunny Boy, he was pulling strands of hay out of his cardboard dispenser and tossing them around the lagomorph lounge like he had never had any anesthesia. He binkied toward me, looking to play, but I just stared into space. He tugged at my pants with his teeth and clawed my feet until I picked him up. There we stood, face to face.

"Everything is going to be fine, Bunny Boy," I whispered, kissing his twittering nose. "I know it will."

As his front paws cupped my cheeks, he licked my nose with a sweetness that, somehow, seemed different.

"I love you so much, little man." I said, looking into his eyes. "I need you, Bunny Boy."

I went to bed earlier than usual. The risk of anesthesia and more invasive surgery weighed heavily on my mind, as it would for the rest of the week.

• • •

The Feast of St. Francis of Assisi, the patron saint of animals, fell just days before Bunny Boy's surgery. I bundled him up in a light blanket and brought him to our church, The Most Blessed Sacrament, to be blessed by Father Mike.

The parking lot behind the church was crowded with cars and pets when we pulled in. There were the usual chocolate and golden Labradors dragging their owners across the lot and at least a dozen brazen lapdogs; longhaired angora cats, tiger-colored kittens, and one Siamese cat; a few hamsters and guinea pigs; and one turtle. And one rabbit—Bunny Boy.

The scene was one of mass pandemonium. Any normal rabbit would have died instantly of a heart attack before receiving the ultimate blessing. Instead, Bunny Boy was cradled in my arms like a baby, perfectly relaxed amid the commotion.

When it was our turn to be blessed, Father Mike asked how old Bunny Boy was and made idle chatter about his fur and size. Like a proud parent, I mentioned that Bunny Boy would pioneer a new treatment at the Animal Medical Center. Father Mike listened intently, then signaled it was time for his blessing. He made the sign of the cross on Bunny Boy's head while he said a short prayer and looked directly into his eyes. Bunny Boy tapped Father Mike's hand with his front right paw as he spoke.

"God will give you the strength to take care of Bunny Boy, Mrs. Laracy."

And I knew God would. Father Mike's calm voice comforted me. It would help me get through a difficult week. I pulled out of the parking lot feeling less anxious and more confident that the surgery would go well.

"You're going to be fine, Bunny Boy. I know that now," I said, reaching over to tickle his ears.

Chapter 17

The stress of Bunny Boy's pending surgery combined with an upper respiratory infection caused another major flare-up in my mixed connective tissue disease. Practically overnight, I felt like I had been run over by a truck. My energy source was completely drained. By the morning of the surgery, it was difficult to walk more than twenty feet without feeling out of breath. Carrying Bunny Boy around had become a chore; he felt so heavy. But I simply had to push through the pain and fatigue for Bunny Boy's sake.

Always striving to be efficient, I had also scheduled an appointment with my rheumatologist Dr. Brown that same day, assuming Bunny Boy would be stable and out of the recovery room by the afternoon. My mother had agreed to accompany me so Ward wouldn't have to miss an important meeting. Mom was remarkable. Nothing stopped her. Not widowhood, not a crippling back or a failed hip replacement. She was always there for her children—and their pets. She also loved New York. When she left her small hometown of Franklin, New Hampshire, in the late 1940s to affiliate as a nurse in Jersey City, Manhattan was her backyard. She was perfectly at home roaming the great metropolis.

We approached the AMC parking lot after sitting in two hours of traffic. My cell phone buzzed as I edged my way forward in the line of cars waiting for the parking attendant. It was Dr. Hess. Bunny Boy's surgery had been canceled. The surgeon who was to operate on Bunny Boy had had a small family emergency.

"I do apologize, Mrs. Laracy. Dr. Irwin assures me that it was just a small emergency and that he can perform the operation tomorrow morning at the same time. He's the most qualified surgeon we have on staff, and Bunny Boy deserves that."

I wanted to bang my head on the steering wheel. It had taken a Herculean effort for me to make the trip. What could I say?

"Can we count on Bunny Boy in the morning?" she asked nicely.

"Yes, we'll be there," I said in my best amicable voice.

I moved my rheumatologist's appointment from two o'clock to eleven. While my mother went to a Starbucks around the corner to pick up some coffee and muffins, Bunny Boy and I waited on the ground floor entrance of the hospital. I was too weak to go for the walk. We hailed a cab around ten thirty and directed the driver to NYU.

"For a moment, I thought that you were holding a cat," said the cab driver in a thick Lebanese accent. "But that's a bunny, and it's big."

"And heavy." I smiled.

"Why all of the hospitals?" he asked.

"This ride is too short for the story."

With Bunny Boy in my arms, I announced myself at the receptionist at Dr. Brown's office. When she replied curtly, Bunny Boy took it upon himself to put an end to her attitude. He hopped onto the counter in his flirtatious style and knocked a pen onto her lap, which only annoyed her more. "I hope your rabbit behaves," she remarked sharply. "You can take a seat and we'll be with you shortly."

My mother and I grabbed two chairs in the crowded, drab lobby. Bunny Boy, his charming and endearing self, relaxed in the crook of my arm. I tickled his belly, and he thrust his thumper paws forward then pulled them backward like he was bench pressing, drawing plenty of attention. My arms were throbbing when I finally asked him if he wanted to get down. He switched from the "cradled infant" position to the "hanging onto my chest for dear life" position, showing no interest in leaving my embrace, provoking a few adoring looks and sweet comments. Eventually, I had no choice.

"Behave, Bunny Boy," I warned, placing him down on the carpet. I should have known better.

Bunny Boy tore around the lobby like one of those crazy mechanical mouses. Patients started lifting their feet and purses. The receptionist let out a shriek and gave me a disapproving look as Bunny Boy binkied toward the exit door and, with one sharp twist of his body, came popcorning back to the table. He stood up on his hind legs and started knocking the magazines onto the floor, one at a time, with his front paws and head. Despite the mess, Mom and I watched as the stress practically lifted from the other patients' faces, to be replaced by smiles as they watched his bunny antics. It was amazing.

Before I could grab my unruly third child, he gamboled several feet in the air and slid across the glass coffee table, landing on a teenager's lap. Bunny Boy started sniffing his crotch like an obnoxious little dog. I ran over, embarrassed, and slung him on my chest, apologizing to the young man. Mom started picking up the magazines, insisting I sit down and rest. "Get him under control," she laughed, "or we'll be thrown out."

Coyly, Bunny Boy burrowed his way down my chest backward and plopped down, snug in the crevice between my legs. With no shame, he sprawled out on his back with his paws up in the air. "He thinks he's a dog," I said, loud enough for the other patients to hear. "Or a baby." By that point, everyone's spirits had been lifted and jovial conversation was flowing.

Dr. Brown walked toward us a few minutes later. He liked to greet his patients in the lobby. "Here's the other member of the family with a screwed-up immune system," I said, jiggling Bunny Boy's belly. Dr. Brown knew all about Bunny Boy.

After the exam, we spoke candidly about the progression of my disease. He recommended more aggressive treatment. Those words sounded familiar and strangely coincidental.

"We can try methotrexate, a chemotherapy drug, or Enbrel, which is one of the newer biologics that block inflammation."

I balked. My fear of starting new medications was real and stemmed back to the early days of my diagnosis. The first rheumatologist I saw prescribed Zoloft at a high dose for pain and not at the dose for depression, and I ended up in the emergency room with a heart rate of 220 and severe deregulation of the central nervous system. It was terrifying enough to influence how I would come to think about and use medication to treat my illnesses. Methotrexate, an immunosuppressant used as chemotherapy, had begun to show great promise in treating rheumatologic diseases by suppressing the immune system; however, it could also be toxic to the liver in the long term and had to be monitored properly. The newer biologics like Enbrel, Humira, and Remicade, a class of immunosuppressants that target a specific part of your information that causes inflammation, were also serious medicines and not without risk. They could cause tuberculosis, multiple sclerosis, and some forms of cancer such as lymphoma and leukemia. For a doctor to start a patient on those types of medications, the benefits had to be weighed carefully against the risks.

"I would like to get some additional blood work before you start anything," said Dr. Brown. "Can you stay around for a few hours?"

It seemed that my time spent dodging more aggressive treatments had finally run out. Reluctantly, I said yes, worrying about my mother's back and hip pain, which she tolerated and disguised so well. And of course, there was Bunny Boy. We had no access to a litter pan.

The nurse came in five minutes later with a shot for my gluteus maximus. She would need to draw blood every half hour for the next two hours to determine if my cortisol levels had returned to normal after having been suppressed from six months of prednisone. If they did, we could start either of the meds.

We relocated to the main lobby to wait. The old New York building looked like it had been built before the turn of the century and had not been renovated since. The walls were a dull gray and the ceiling was stained, with numerous tiles missing. A security guard inside of a small glass cubicle greeted visitors as they came in. When there was a lull, he walked over.

"I'm not sure I've ever seen somebody traveling with a bunny. Not even in New York." He rubbed Bunny Boy's head with his knuckles. His name was LeRoy, and his southern drawl and proper demeanor were welcoming and charming. LeRoy hung around and chatted with us until I went in for my next shot. He was intrigued by Bunny Boy and thought his ten grandchildren—five girls and five boys—would love him.

By the time I returned to the lobby, it was time for lunch. According to LeRoy, there were no food establishments within walking distance except for the bodega across the street.

"They have great Chinese food, if you like that kind of thing."

I looked outside. It was pouring rain.

"I'll be happy to lend you one of those fine umbrellas over yonder!" He brought us one of the umbrellas from the stand next to his cubicle. "I'd be mighty pleased if you would leave the bunny with me while you all go and get yourselves some lunch."

How could we refuse his offer? Plus, Bunny Boy would go to anyone, just like Julie had as a baby.

When I saw the vast array of Cantonese items at the buffet, I knew it was worth the effort it took for me to walk over. We returned with two Styrofoam containers of delicacies to find Bunny Boy propped on LeRoy's knees.

"He's quite an amicable fellow," said Leroy, winking at us.

I was biting into a crisp piece of stir-fried broccoli, Bunny Boy on my lap, when my mom motioned for me to look up. An incredibly handsome and sophisticated gentleman had just walked in. He wore a Burberry raincoat and held a Davek umbrella. He walked with a smooth, wide stride, and then stopped abruptly when he saw us out of the corner of his eye. It was difficult to see the expression on his face.

"Maybe he's flirting with you, honey!" my mom said. More than likely, he was just surprised to see us having lunch with a bunny!

As he approached our bench with a distinct air of confidence, he raised his eyebrows in an awkward sort of way and looked me over again. Uncomfortably. Bunny Boy bolted upright on my lap, eying the intruder.

"You must be kidding," he snarled. "You're eating in the foyer of my apartment building." My temper flared, and I signaled to my mother in a way that said, "Let me handle this."

"We're so sorry," I began, in my kindest, most nauseating voice possible. "My mother and I were hungry. I'm having blood drawn every half hour by Dr. Brown, which doesn't leave us enough time to venture out to a restaurant, so LeRoy recommended we get some food across the street.

Besides the fact, I feel quite sick. We're going to be here for two more hours."

He came closer, and his mean look startled me. But I continued my sweet talk, fully hoping to shame him for his insensitivity. "Perhaps we could go outside in the rain and sit on the curb and have our lunch if you would like?"

"Please do," he barked. My mother was halfway off the bench in protest of his ghastly manners, but she settled back down when I put my arm out to block her like a gate. Now it was my turn to bark. I covered Bunny Boy's ears and spit out more four-letter expletives than Al Pacino had in *Scarface*. My mother looked at me in disbelief, as if she had no idea who I was. The vulgar language was uncharacteristic of me. I had clearly been suffering from blood loss. He returned some verbal fire. Suddenly, Bunny Boy lunged forward with his front paws and snarled angrily, nearly falling onto the ground, and the man fled for the elevator, not looking back. Mom stared at Bunny Boy in the same way she had looked at me just moments before. Neither one of us had any idea Bunny Boy could make such an aggressive sound. It was worse than the day he challenged the squirrel. And the fact that he had detected hostility and seemed to want to protect us was simply unbelievable.

LeRoy walked over and shook my hand. "There are probably a half a dozen folks in this building who would love to do what you just did!"

Manhattan had finally met Bunny Boy!

• • •

We made the second trek into New York City the following morning without incident. Bunny Boy clung to Dr. Hess's shoulder, looking back at me, as she walked down the hallway toward the operating room. I could tell he was frightened. So was I. A Ziploc bag containing my two favorite prayer cards—one specifically for animals and another to St. Francis—were tucked safely in her jacket pocket. I needed the prayer cards to be near Bunny Boy while he was in surgery. Once they disappeared, I huddled in the warm embrace of my mother. I often wondered if I would have had a similar relationship with my father had he lived long enough to know me as a grown woman.

By noon, Bunny Boy was in recovery. I had chewed most of my cuticles and stared at the colorful jungle mural on the far wall of the lobby, second-guessing my decision. Now that Bunny Boy had made it through the anesthesia, I felt as if a heavy load had been lifted off my shoulders.

When Dr. Hess came for us, I went to stand up, and my joint pain was almost unbearable. Everything around me began to spin. The colors in the mural melded together like a kaleidoscope and the hallway to the recovery room seemed to be narrowing as we walked down to see Bunny Boy.

"The surgery went well, Mrs. Laracy," Dr. Hess reassured me, wrapping her arm around my shoulder. "Bunny Boy is resting comfortably. You can relax a little now."

"Thank you," was all I managed to say.

"Are you okay? You look a little pale."

My mother quickly answered for me. "She's fine now."

We walked into the unit, past many pets in small incubator-style containers. I looked at them uneasily. They all belonged to someone who loved them. A surgical tech walked over, holding Bunny Boy. He was swaddled in a yellow towel like an infant. His nose and whiskers were perfectly still, and his eyes were covered with a gel-like substance. I leaned down and kissed his soft cheek and dry nose.

"Mommy loves you very much, Bunny Boy. You're so strong."

Instantly, Bunny Boy's whiskers began to flutter every so slightly and his nose began to twitter. All of my angst and worry disappeared. My boy had made it through the surgery. And he had done his part to help veterinary research.

"Your mutual affection for each other is captivating," said Dr. Hess, with a genuineness that told me she meant it. Then she gave us some troubling news. She had found two small abscesses in Bunny Boy's hocks. They were most likely caused by the same strain of bacteria that was in his jaw abscess.

"I will show you how to irrigate and bandage these wounds. This is critical, so please watch closely."

She unwrapped the towel and then the two separate layers of bandages on Bunny Boy's hind legs. Bunny Boy began to stir. I could see two small holes in the center of his hocks where the fur had been shaved.

"This must be done every day, religiously, for six weeks to prevent the infection from entering the bone." Dr. Hess drew a light blue fluid up into a small syringe and injected it into the wounds where the pus had been. The technician held onto Bunny Boy firmly as he squirmed. It was difficult for me to watch. It was apparent that his hocks were painful. Once the wounds were irrigated, she applied a generous amount of antibiotic cream and a soft pad covering, and together they bandaged his legs with gauze and a colorful rubber wrapping. His legs were immobilized at a right angle. I wondered how he would hop around—maybe he couldn't.

"Bunny Boy will also need daily penicillin shots and an oral antibiotic for six weeks. And please do not forget to do the hot compresses on his jaw. These tubes will drain easier if the fluid isn't thick."

My eyes darted from his hocks to his jaw, which was swollen and beginning to turn black and blue. It was overwhelming. I wanted to say, "Wait, slow down. This is too much to process so quickly."

My mom, the nurse, jumped right in. "You can handle this, Nance. We can handle this."

Of course I could. And I would.

"On a positive note, Bunny Boy's a pioneer!" said Dr. Hess. "He's one of the first rabbits to have the antibiotics beads implanted during a debridement. That's the lump that you see here." She pointed to his jaw.

Dr. Irwin, the surgeon, had also removed some scar tissue from Bunny Boy's previous surgery and shaved a piece of his jawbone in case the infection had spread into the bone.

"We'd like to use Bunny Boy's records for an educational seminar next month with our incoming veterinary residents, if that's alright with you?" she asked. "Bunny Boy's records may be used worldwide for research purposes as well. We are a prominent teaching animal hospital."

I couldn't have been prouder of Bunny Boy. In a strange way, it was a triumphant moment for him.

Another would be when the groundbreaking research he had been a part of would begin to be used on humans.

I walked out of the hospital feeling like a supply clerk for Doctors Without Borders. Bunny Boy's "go home" bag was filled with a rainbow selection of elastic bandages, gauze bandages for his paws, and several different medications, each with their separate dosing instructions. Pre-filled penicillin injections. Pain medication. Antibacterial cream. Oral antibiotics. The itemized bill trailed out of the bag. There was also a large box of critical care food—Bunny Boy's favorite health food. I assumed based on the size of the box that I would be hand-feeding Bunny Boy for a while.

As Mom pulled out of the parking garage with my car, she looked over at me. Bunny Boy was resting comfortably in my arms, reswaddled. "You wanted a third baby, honey," she said gently.

"Yes I did, Mom."

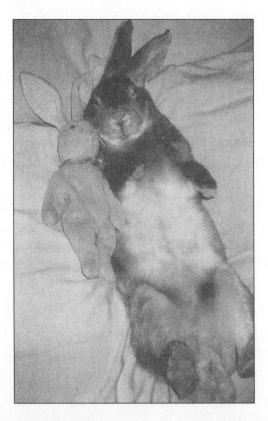

Chapter 18

Bunny Boy's daily regimen of care became a family affair. It was a special bonding time for the five of us. Our infamous junk drawer, once full of spare keys, miscellaneous office supplies, emery boards, old batteries, thumbtacks, and god knows what else, was now full of neatly organized medical supplies. Julie was in charge of keeping the inventory up to date. When the bandages got low, we went to see our friends at the Franklin Lakes Animal Hospital with Bunny Boy in tow, his hocks wrapped in different colored bandages each visit to keep him and me from getting bored. By the fourth week, Donna, one of the technicians at the hospital, said as she handed us our bag, "I added some fluorescent colors and patterns such as stars or stripes to our weekly supply order."

I took great care to keep a sterile environment. Through trial and error, we figured out how to wrap the perfect bandage. Once, we wrapped the bandage too tightly, and within half an hour, Bunny Boy's toes were so swollen they looked like they would explode. Others were too loose, and our Houdini bunny deftly pried them off in one piece.

As we approached the holiday season, the variety of color choices for the bandages became a playful issue of contention among the kids and me.

"Let's wrap one hock in red and one in green for Christmas," I suggested in mid-November, violating the house rule that the Christmas season could not begin before the day after Thanksgiving. Chris mumbled something that sounded like, "She's ridiculous!"

"I won't play Christmas music until December 5 instead of Black Friday, if you let me put on the red and green bandages on Bunny Boy," I told him.

"It's a great deal, kids!" exclaimed Ward. "As your attorney, I'm telling you to take the plea bargain."

The Christmas season started officially on Thanksgiving at our house and ended on January 6, during the Feast of the Epiphany, otherwise known as "Little Christmas." Seasonal tunes played around the clock on the radio in the kitchen or in the car while I drove Julie and Chris to their activities. Ward and the children were not fans of Christmas music. It was sheer torture for them to hear Dominick the Donkey clop or Andy Williams whine about not being home for Christmas. Updated Christmas gift lists were the only reason Julie and Chris complied with my request.

The holidays flew by, bringing their usual joy, excitement and stress. By the time Little Christmas came around, even I was tired of hearing Christmas music and looking at the holiday clutter. And Ward was tired of taking the trash out to the garage. We had accumulated enough medical waste to fill our own barge, but it was worth all the effort to see Bunny Boy's jaw and hocks heal wonderfully and for the abscesses to be gone. Now, we could only just pray and rely on modern veterinary medicine. It had been sad to see Bunny Boy grounded for a few weeks, though it didn't seem to bother him at all. Watching him popcorn and leap up onto the sofa again was a welcome sight. Much to Dr. Hess's surprise, Bunny Boy returned to eating his food pellets three days after the surgery. Strangely, however, he showed no interest in grazing on hay as the weeks passed. We soon discovered that his jaw had been misaligned from the surgery. That, combined with his misaligned teeth, made it impossible for him to eat hay, which would cause another host of problems. Bunny Boy would need to have his front teeth—top and bottom—trimmed every two weeks for the remainder of his life and his molars trimmed twice a year.

The remainder of the winter was kind to us. We had very little snow, intermittent bursts of 50° weather, and plenty of sunshine. By some small miracle, I was also able to put off starting methotrexate or Enbrel yet again when a last-ditch titration of steroids helped to stabilize me. I felt like I had dodged a bullet.

• • •

Life was passing by too quickly, and my children were growing up in front of my eyes.

Julie was enjoying communicating with her friends on Facebook and dancing in her bedroom while listening to music on her iPod until the wee hours of the night. Sometimes softly, sometimes not so softly. On work nights, Ward would lower the boom. "You dance, you die." Chris had grown over three inches and was in fantastic shape from rigorous workouts at the gym with his father. He moved like a panther and rebounded like Kobe Bryant. But he had some stiff competition—Bunny Boy. Our adorable rabbit could binky almost four feet into the air—and he was still gaining yardage. I called him the flying miracle bunny. Bunny Boy's incredible resilience, happy-go-lucky spirit, and will to survive were infectious. He had brought such happiness to our home. But Chris still believed there was more in store for Bunny Boy.

It was a clear, cool spring day. The wall of fuchsia and white azaleas on the corner of the property was at peak growth, fragrant and colorful. The petals from the cherry trees had formed a soft pink and white blanket along the front porch. On windy days, the petals swirled across the grass like feathers.

Chris came barreling through the front door looking for Bunny Boy. Loudly, he announced that the new neighbor diagonally across the street, whom I had yet to meet, had a two-year-old girl and two bunnies. Like a Stepford Wife, I had hoped to bring over my versions of the classic Jell-O mold and Lee Bailey's decadent chocolate brownies once the moving truck unloaded, but for various reasons I had yet to welcome the new neighbors. Chris insisted we bring Bunny Boy right over.

With a look of mischief in his eyes, Chris nudged Bunny Boy awake. "Bunny Boy can have play dates, Mom! They have a huge outdoor playground!"

The idea of showing off Bunny Boy to another bunny owner excited me, though Chris and I were not on the same page regarding unleashing Bunny Boy into an outdoor playground.

Bunny Boy, who had just napped, started racing around like a contestant in the Indy 500. Julie ran down the stairs; she had overheard the phrase "two-year-old" and was thinking immediately about the babysitting opportunity. Julie had recently become our second little entrepreneur. She took full advantage of her love for young children and had spent the previous summer working as a day camp counselor, teaching seven-year-olds tennis in the evenings, while babysitting on weekends. Suddenly, she had disposable income.

"I'll go with you," she said exuberantly, surprising Chris. "Maybe I can become their babysitter."

We rang the neighbor's bell. No one answered. Chris brought us around to the backyard, where we quickly found Ivy, the owner, sitting in a white wooden rocking chair reading *The Hungry Caterpillar* to her daughter, Ivanna. Ivy was tall, her straight chestnut-brown hair cropped just below her ears. She had large, round blue eyes. Ivanna had luscious brown curls, blue eyes like her mother, and a toothless smile.

I kept the introductions brief, emphasizing the babysitter card. Bunny Boy was nestled in Julie's right arm with his belly facing forward in what I liked to call the "Titanic" position, because he reminded me of Rose as she waited to be sketched by Jack. Ivanna reached over and touched Bunny Boy's head ever so gently.

"Wook. Boo boo."

"Yes, it's a bunny,'" said Ivy, translating for her daughter. "We could never carry our bunnies that way, Nancy," she remarked, as if envious of the way Julie was holding Bunny Boy.

"He's an indoor bunny who thinks he's my baby," I explained.

We decided to move to the front gardens instead, since the elaborate playpen in the backyard was temporarily off limits as it had recently been sprayed with lawn chemicals. Chris was heartily disappointed. Ivy opened the hutch, retrieved Isabella and Scout, and walked us around to the front gardens. The gardens at the front of the house, I already knew, were spectacular. I admired them almost every day. The previous owner had planted and maintained a perennial garden that was the envy of the entire neighborhood. She was the only neighbor with full sunlight on her yard from dawn until dusk.

The sun was blazing that afternoon. The stars must have been in alignment. I was feeling particularly energetic and almost pain-free from two steroid shots the doctor had injected into my lower back three days before, a new treatment we were trying intermittently to control my pain. I plopped Bunny Boy down in the middle of the bulbous fuchsia peonies. The scent of the flowers was dreamy. Julie watched out of the corner of her eye while she swung Ivanna around on the grass, not wasting any time securing her next babysitting job.

Bunny Boy sniffed the different leaves and wispy flowers, gently nibbling at their tips. Then he started digging at the roots of the plants, tossing dirt up into the air. A butterfly fluttered close, almost touching his tail. He settled back on his haunches and gazed at the butterfly, whose wings were the color of a sunflower. Bunny Boy's satin fur glistened in the sunlight; his whiskers fluttered like the butterfly. Our prince looked radiant.

Then, he noticed Ivy's bunnies. Scout, a black Lionhead with a classic, light, fluffy mane and short ears, had taken a liking to Chris. Isabella, with charcoal-gray fur and white on one side of her face, was striking. Bunny Boy kicked up his hind legs and binkied in Isabella's direction, landing in front of her with a bounce. Then he did the cutest thing and pranced by her, the way he had the first time he used his litter pan successfully. I think he was flirting. He changed direction and gamboled into the air, getting a huge amount of air time, and landed in front of her a second time, stopping to stare into her deep green eyes. I thought of Thumper from the movie *Bambi*, who was always bouncing and ending up somewhere he didn't belong.

We all watched the budding romance as it unfolded. Bunny Boy sniffed the white side of Isabella's face and her hind legs. Isabella flipped her body sharply, as if initially rejecting his advances, but landing such that once again they were face to face. I thought it was intriguing that Scout, the male rabbit, showed no interest in Bunny Boy. Bunny Boy and Isabella nudged each other's faces for a few moments, as if introducing themselves. Then they began to frolic in the grass, almost skimming across the tops of the soft green blades. They chased each other around flowers and binkied in and out of the trees until they collapsed from exhaustion. They nestled together, bodies almost attached, and groomed each other delicately like two bunnies falling in love. As difficult as it was for me to admit, I had never seen Bunny Boy so happy.

When we finally walked home, schoolwork was the last thing on the children's minds. We were too busy chattering about our next visit to the new neighbors. Bunny Boy had a rabbit playmate now, and Julie had sparked up a friendship with Ivy and Ivanna that would turn out to be a lucrative financial arrangement. And Chris had clearly met his match in Scout.

• • •

It was an emotional time for me. A month later, Julie graduated middle school, and Chris graduated fifth grade a few days after. At Julie's graduation, I reached for Ward's hand as I sat looking up at the podium, thinking, *Where had the years gone? The sandboxes and swings? The day-trips to the local farm or petting zoo?* Julie walked up proudly for her diploma, wearing her rainbow-sherbet-pastel-colored gown and an updo fit for a princess. Chris's ceremony was small but no less significant. We were all so proud. And so was Bunny Boy. There had been a few not-so-serious discussions as to whether or not we could bring him to the actual graduations! Finally, Julie, who always prided herself on being different, was confirmed Julianne Marie "St. Cloud" Laracy at the end of June, despite her earlier objections to partake in the sacrament of confirmation.

Mid-summer, Bunny Boy's fairy tale romance came to an abrupt end. A coyote had killed a darling puppy while she was out in her yard. It was tragic; just the thought of it made me shudder. I knew it wasn't safe to allow Bunny Boy outside any longer.

"Bunny Boy will just have to snuggle with you on your bed, Nance," said Ward. "And he can dream of Isabella." He winked.

"Or, we can get him his own bunny playmate," Chris chimed in without a moment's hesitation. Pretending not to hear him, I started folding a load of laundry. In his typical, well-thought-out manner, Chris started quoting statistics from published studies on the Internet about the advantages of bunnies cohabitating. And there were many. I listened and nodded in acknowledgment and kept folding clothes. He began helping with his own T-shirts, desperate and determined to keep me engaged.

"Mom, you aren't taking this seriously. Bunny Boy needs and wants a playmate."

Neither Ward nor I wanted another bunny.

"Let's talk to your father," I suggested, hoping to settle the matter once and for all.

Ward was in the middle of a phone conversation with his brother, Gregory.

"It's still cheaper than college tuition," I heard Ward say, to which Gregory replied, "Just make a pot of stew!" His voice was loud enough for me to hear.

I shrieked playfully and gave Ward a dirty look. I had gotten the gist of what they were talking about even before I'd heard Gregory's last comment. I could see Ward's lawyer mind working overtime on his reply.

"I was just telling Gregory about Bunny Boy's surgery, Nance. Specifically, how much it cost."

In a fake huff, I scooped up Bunny Boy and placed him on Ward's lap. "Just make a pot of stew!" I repeated.

"Come on, Nance. It was all a big joke. Gregory knows how much Bunny Boy means to all of us. But most people don't realize what wonderful pets bunnies can make!" I could tell he also wanted to say, "expensive pets."

Ward decided to come clean. "I told him Bunny Boy was your third child. And that his medical bills were still a lot cheaper than four years of college."

"Anything else?"

"I may have mentioned how you tell Bunny Boy you love him more than life itself . . ." he trailed off.

Chris and I burst into laughter. We ran over and gave Ward and Bunny Boy a big hug. "We love you, Bunny Boy," I said, giving him noogies. "And I love you too, honey," I said sneakily to Ward.

Chapter 19

At a time when I felt my teenaged Julie naturally slipping away, suddenly we had a new common bond that brought us closer.

High school was due to start in only six weeks, and Julie had an announcement.

"Mom, I'd like to try out for the high school tennis team." She said it with the conviction of someone who had played years of tennis, not someone who only played socially on Friday afternoons during middle school. Our suburban town of Franklin Lakes was one of the top three competitive tennis towns in New Jersey. Most children started swinging a racket by the age of three, many times on the courts built in their own backyards. Tennis lessons might just as well have been part of the school curriculum. But Ward and I thought Julie must be kidding.

In second grade, Julie had given up basketball and soccer, and we thought—at least at the time—that she didn't have the fire in her belly to compete. "Oh no, I can't take the ball away from her," she told her basketball coach, casting a look of great empathy toward her opponent. "She'll get too upset." Another time, she sat on the soccer field during a game and chatted it up with a girlfriend while the ball was in play on the other end of the field. "Honey, get back in the game," I mouthed, waving my hands, trying to get her attention. As parents of the millennial generation, we hadn't dared discourage our little muffin from trying any sport, lest we damage her self-esteem.

And so Julie's most recent change of heart took us by pleasant surprise. Just five weeks of intense lessons at our tennis club and the right attitude turned up a hidden star. Our five-foot-tall, one-hundred-pound daughter, quickly nicknamed "The Wall" or "Down-the-Line Laracy" by her team, played junior varsity tennis as a freshman in a very competitive district, challenging the most seasoned players, even those with twice her height and girth. She would stroll onto the court with an air of confidence I would have killed for.

Julie would start each match with a winning smile and a very weak handshake.

"Good luck," she would say, barely audible, instilling a false of sense of confidence in her opponents, though not intentional. To their shock, usually within a half hour, they would come running to the fence breathless and frustrated, saying to their coach, "What do I do now? She hits everything back."

Julie rendered her opponents exhausted. Her strategy early in the season was simply to wear down her opponents. Needless to say, we were all enjoying the rebirth of Julie's athletic career. Her dynamic tennis matches became the highlight of the fall, which also included Chris's soccer season.

Bunny Boy would usually be at the games to watch the slaughter—weather permitting. If it was hotter than eighty degrees, he remained behind. Heat stroke is very common in rabbits. When Bunny Boy was there, we would watch Julie from my camping chair. He would sit on my lap in his "high alert—I'm happy" stance and stare at the court, seemingly interested in what was going on. Bunny Boy taught me you could be an enthusiastic fan by quietly using positive body language—just like the uppity rituals of tennis, which were a new experience. I was used to Chris's contact sports, where pretty much anything went. Bullhorns and whistles were background noise. Ward was known to run up and down the sidelines on the soccer field or basketball court, pumping up Chris, while I screamed from the bleachers. At least some things still stayed the same. When Ward was able to come to Julie's afternoon matches, he would pace behind the bleachers and shake his head. "I'm far less tense when I'm working on a multimillion-dollar deal, for Pete's sake."

I soon earned my "team mom" status, traveling throughout the state to Julie's matches and hosting pasta parties, complete with a brilliant cake for dessert—a fluorescent-yellow iced tennis ball designed by our local bakery. I was playfully chastised by the coach for bringing homemade donuts as the girls' snacks early in the season instead of fruit and granola bars. But I got back in her good graces by listening to stories about "Harry," her dwarf bunny, and designing a knock-'em-dead poster for the state championships. For the first time in the history of the high school, the girls' tennis team made it to the state championships. I was enjoying living vicariously through my talented teenage daughter. And so was Bunny Boy, who finally had the chance to become a mascot for Julie's tennis team—at least in her mind and mine.

• • •

By mid-October, autumn was in full bloom. Fall in the northeast is a spectacle of nature. The fiery blaze of colors from the trees ranges in hues from red to gold, creating a magnificent backdrop for the many lakes and quaint towns. But fall also means traffic jams along most of the northeast coast, and homeowners have to rake or blow leaves constantly to keep their lawns pristine.

I, too, had a new love-hate relationship with autumn. I dreaded the increase in my pain level. Fibromyalgia patients suffer tremendously from barometric pressure swings. Sudden changes in temperature, characteristic of the spring and fall, wreak havoc on our bodies. But I loved the changing landscape as the summer palettes of pink and purple flowers withered away and were replaced by the bright orange, red, and yellow leaves from the majestic deciduous trees that define the Bergen County suburbs. I welcomed the lack of humidity and the slightly cooler temperatures. After a long, hot summer, I looked forward to putting on a sweatshirt and curling up with a good book and a cup of hot tea or relaxing in our outdoor Jacuzzi with the family, chatting and stargazing.

We had scheduled a complete overhaul of our family room, Bunny Boy's primary place of residence, for October 25. The demolition date crept up on us overnight and we were still scrambling to empty out cluttered bookcases and closets to vacate the lagomorph lounge. Except for

Bunny Boy. He was boycotting the whole project, stretched out on the sofa in a "leave me alone, I'm chilling" position. Thirty minutes into the project, Julie and Chris were already bickering over who had done the most work, and Ward was designating anything that wasn't nailed down to the floors or walls as garbage.

When it came time to tackle the electronic equipment, tensions were high. Ward and Chris struggled to remove the oversized vintage television from the sixties-style bookcase and began maneuvering it on the landing. That got Bunny Boy's attention. Suddenly, he was nosing around at their feet. It was only when they tripped on the short staircase leading down into the kitchen—crashing into the wall and nearly toppling down head-first—that Bunny Boy showed an urgency to relocate. He tore back into the room then out again, confused as to what was the best escape route. He overshot the landing and skidded between the guys' legs.

"Get him out of the way!" Ward yelled. "We're all going to get hurt."

I jumped up and tried to grab him as he struggled to get his bearings, but he clawed frantically on each slippery hardwood step and crashed down onto the hard, ceramic kitchen tile. I ran downstairs. Bunny Boy was sitting at the bottom of the stairs, swiping at his jaw with his right paw and sneezing. Ward and Chris sat on the stairs with the television on their lap, breathing heavily.

I lifted Bunny Boy up gently, supporting his hind legs in case they were injured. I checked his entire jawbone, which was my first concern. He swatted me with his paw, sneezed again, then leapt out of my arms and popcorned playfully toward Julie who was taking a "Red Bull break."

"Bunny Boy seems fine, but Chris and I hurt our arms," Ward said. "Just get Bunny Boy out of the way."

I locked Bunny Boy in his fictitious favorite bathroom to get him out of the danger zone.

Soon, the family room looked like burglars had ransacked it. Wires hung from behind bookcases. Drawers were pulled halfway out. Empty baskets were flipped over. The boys carried out the computer and printer while Julie and I tossed any final items into baskets for the garbage and swept up. Given the deadline, the Laracy family had come through.

When I opened the bathroom door to let Bunny Boy out, I let out a bloodcurdling scream. Bunny Boy was sitting upright on the toilet in a pool of blood, licking his paws. The bathroom looked like a crime scene. Blood was splattered all over the moldings. The toilet. The walls. And the marble floor. Careful not to slip, I edged my way slowly toward him, my heart racing. Fear swept through me. Within seconds, the whole family was squeezed into the tiny bathroom trying to assess Bunny Boy's injuries. I grabbed a towel and gently wiped his head, ears, face, and body, searching for the origin of the blood. Strangely, Bunny Boy seemed to enjoy the rub down. His big ears were in the "happy" position and his nose was twittering at a normal pace. I lifted him up to check his underside, assuming the worst. Then I saw it.

"It's a ripped nail!" I announced, like I had just delivered a baby. The stress evaporated from my body. Bunny Boy must have torn one of his nails on his right front paw when he slid down the stairs. It was hanging on by a thread. I couldn't imagine that such an injury could produce so much blood. He looked up at me as if to say, "Don't sweat the small stuff," and resumed his licking.

"Bunny Boy's a real character, isn't he?" said Chris.

"We'll never be bored as long as he's in the house," Ward joked.

Then his tone quickly changed to one of concern. "What's this?"

In case the bathroom wasn't enough of a disaster, Ward had noticed a puddle of urine behind the toilet.

"It's his urine. The fall probably frightened him."

"It's more than a male sprinkle, Dad. Let's see if Bunny Boy gets in trouble like we do!" Chris joked, waiting for me to chastise our rabbit.

But I was not convinced Bunny Boy had peed out of fear. He had been through much worse. He had never had another bladder accident since he was a kit. My motherly instincts told me he might have a bladder infection.

I phoned Dr. Welch first thing the next morning. Neither suspicion of a bladder infection nor a torn nail constituted an emergency. We had treated more serious ailments and bandaged a lot more than a torn nail on Bunny Boy. Dr. Welch was out on maternity leave, having given birth to twins. Her partner, Dr. Kozak, agreed to see us that afternoon.

Dr. Kozak was young, like Dr. Welch, with a nice temperament, but she claimed not to be an exotics expert, though she knew enough about rabbits.

"From everything I've heard, this little guy has taught Cheryl that some rabbits are stronger and more resilient than what she learned in medical school," said Dr. Kozak, fiddling with her stethoscope. "She believes Bunny Boy's heart has grown stronger because he is loved so much."

"Why, thank you," I replied in gratitude. "I would like to think so."

"So, what makes you think Bunny Boy has a bladder infection, Mrs. Laracy?"

"I know Bunny Boy almost as well as I know my children. But for a few isolated slip-ups when he was a kit, Bunny Boy has had complete control over his bladder. Yesterday he peed in the bathroom, not in his litter pan."

"What happened to his paw?"

"He slid down a flight of stairs and hurt his nail. We're lucky that's all that happened to him."

She took a close look, then cleaned and rebandaged his paw. "It's nothing to worry about."

Bunny Boy licked her hand and lightly swatted her cheek when she leaned down with her stethoscope to listen to his heart. "I see what Dr. Welch means." She smiled. "He's very sweet and cooperative."

She reached under Bunny Boy's butt, squeezed his bladder, and then opened the cabinet above the exam table and took out a test strip. "This will be our answer." She dipped the stick into the pool of urine on the paper lining of the table.

Dr. Kozak returned ten minutes later, holding the results. With a twinkle in her eye she said, "You have a very intuitive mommy, Bunny Boy. You have a bladder infection."

She handed me a prescription for an antibiotic cream for the torn nail, as well as Baytril, an oral antibiotic for the bladder infection.

"Nice to have met you both." She reached her hand out to shake mine. "Bunny Boy is lucky to have you as his owner. Sadly, we don't see rabbits getting the best care. Owners give up on them quickly, unfortunately."

"The luck of the bunny is how we found each other," I said. "And some divine intervention."

Chapter 20

Shortly after his bladder infection, Bunny Boy contracted "snuffles," an upper respiratory infection from the bacteria Pasteurella, which is common in rabbits and very resistant to antibiotic treatment. The bacteria had caused a systemic infection in Bunny Boy, one that he would battle for the rest of his life.

Around the same time, a serious influenza virus struck our town early in the new school year. Flu shots had just become available. At one point, so many children were absent from the middle school that they considered closing for a day or two.

The children and Ward got sick first. For almost three weeks, I went into nursing mode, knowing fully how dangerous it might be if I got the flu. I washed my hands so much they became chapped and turned bright pink. "When people are sick, that's when they need you," my mom would always tell me, whether she was talking about complete strangers or family members.

When I finally got the respiratory influenza, Ward and the children had thankfully recovered. I was so sick I barely left my bed for days. While the fever subsided after a week, the cough continued for close to a month and some old but familiar symptoms returned with a vengeance. My immune system refused to shut down like a normal person's and reactivated some of my dormant viruses, namely parvovirus B-19. It had been ten years since my life had been turned upside down by that virus.

I met with Dr. Pasik, who had overseen my first round of intravenous gamma globulin many years back when I was first diagnosed. After extensive blood work, DNA PCR testing, and medical paperwork, Ward drove me to Princeton, New Jersey, to meet with a committee of physicians from our insurance company who would decide whether or not I could receive the treatment. I was approved before we made it back to our car, despite the fact that there was a worldwide shortage of the product. Intravenous gamma globulin is a blood transfer product that is made up of hundreds of people's antibodies to infections that can help the compromised immune system of the patient to fight back. But mad cow disease had just been discovered in Europe, and the vials of IV gamma globulin in circulation had not been screened for it and were possibly contaminated. Every vial was pulled off the market. It takes about nine months to make a new supply, and so until more IV gamma globulin became available, doctors and insurance companies used extreme caution, prescribing it on a severity of need basis. Each infusion was eleven thousand dollars, and I would need six treatments, once a month.

The timing could not have been worse. Ward had recently been appointed to sit on the board of directors for one of his largest clients, and we had proudly offered to host a holiday party for the executives and their spouses. We had both assumed the renovation of the family room would be finished in time, which was a pipe dream.

Julie wanted to go with me for my first IV infusion at the Carol Simon Cancer in Morristown. When she and Chris were younger, I went to great lengths to shield them from the more serious aspects of my illness. But as they grew up and matured, I decided that having them know I was sick was not necessarily a bad thing; it could also teach them to be more compassionate, caring human beings. Living with joint and muscle pain around the clock was disheartening and frustrating, and I needed their patience, much like my mother needed ours when I was growing up. When my mother lost twenty-five pounds from the stress of working as a nurse and caring for Dad, the house, and us, we took on more household responsibilities and tried to be there for her emotionally. Having a sick father was challenging. Though Dad rarely looked sick, we knew that his heart and body were struggling on the inside. We did our best to treat him with love and kindness even on the days when he was grumpy. Without prompting from my mother, we rearranged our busy schedules to make sure Dad was never left alone. He would not have survived his first heart attack if someone had not been home to call for help.

And now, Julie was there for me. I was proud and thankful to have her company for what would be a long, arduous, uncomfortable day.

Ward dropped us off at the center around nine in the morning. A volunteer escorted us upstairs to the third floor. Leather recliners lined the perimeter of the treatment room. Large windows on the north side of the building allowed plenty of sun to pour in, and soothing artwork—ocean scenes and garden landscapes—hung on the sage-green walls. Brightly colored and striped afghans were folded neatly on the vacant chairs, and there was a small coffee bar in a corner. Despite the welcoming accoutrements, it was hard to overlook the dreadfully ill-looking patients and all of the medical equipment.

A burly nurse, carrying my million-dollar medicine, walked us over to chair number nine. "Did you take your prednisone this morning?" she asked while she set up her supplies.

"I did."

In this treatment, the steroids were supposed to suppress my immune system enough to allow my body to accept the antibodies to the many viruses and bacteria that make up gamma globulin. Prednisone also decreased the chance of me going into anaphylactic shock, a possible effect of the treatment. There was nothing about anaphylactic shock that I didn't understand or fear. At times, it could be fatal.

With very little effort, the nurse found my veins. I settled into my chair, wrapped in my comfy afghan, Julie by my side. Every fifteen minutes, the nurse would come over and check my blood pressure and temperature and ask me if there was anything I needed. A slight rise in blood pressure and body temperature is expected during the course of the treatment, but anything more than slight would be a concern.

About an hour into the infusion, my temperature went up to 100 degrees, which felt like a real fever compared to my average body temperature of around 97. A low body temperature is typical of many people suffering from autoimmune diseases. I asked for an extra blanket and some chamomile tea to ward off the chill deep in my bones. By that point, the muscle cramps and chest pain were becoming uncomfortable. Julie switched off the television, showing concern.

"It's completely normal, Jules," I said, trying to reassure her that I was fine. "When you or Chris have an infection, you run a fever, right?"

"Uh huh," she said, in a way that told me she wasn't convinced.

"Your immune system is fighting off the infection and produces certain chemicals that raise your temperature. Right now, my body's natural response is to fight off the antibodies in that small bottle." I pointed to the IV pole. "It's the same concept."

She nodded slowly as if she understood. If she was pretending, I didn't pick up on it. Hoping to change the topic, I barged in on the conversation between the two women to my right.

"I couldn't help but overhear you have a little Westie," I said. One woman wore a brightly colored bandana tied around her bald head. She didn't have eyebrows or eyelashes. I assumed she was undergoing chemotherapy. The other woman, who I later found out had lupus, was receiving methotrexate, which I was very familiar with.

"But she's no ordinary Westie!" Jennifer, the woman with the bandana, exclaimed, almost bouncing up in her recliner. Boy, did her tone sound familiar! She whipped her billfold out of her purse, which was full of adorable pictures of Biscuit, her once-drawn face suddenly lit up with a smile. For the next half hour, we listened to one endearing, silly story after another about Biscuit, the not-so-ordinary Westie.

"I have a not-so-ordinary rabbit," I said finally, when there was a significant lull in the conversation.

"OMG—don't get my mother started on our rabbit," said Julie. I saw their puzzled looks.

"*Oh-em-gee* means *oh my god*," I explained to them. "It's teen language."

Lacking a billfold to unleash, I reached for my cell phone. My wallpaper featured Bunny Boy wearing his Santa hat.

"Bunny Boy has free run of our house and loves riding on the front seat of the car. He also loves playing poker with the family."

Now that I had started, it was hard to stop. "He's the love of my life," I sighed, wrapping the blanket tighter around my chilled body.

"Bunny Boy licks me and kisses me on the lips," I continued, shamelessly. I couldn't help myself. When it came to Bunny Boy and my children, I felt happiness down to my soul. "And he purrs like a cat."

Julie looked at me with great trepidation and slouched down in her chair, as if she could sense what I was about to say next.

"When he gets too excited, he sprays me," I blurted out. "He won't spray anyone else."

"Mooooom!" Julie shrieked. "TMI!"

"That means *too much information*," I translated, realizing I had gone too far. There was an awkward silence.

"He sprays you with what?" came the obvious question.

"Urine," I whispered. If the women were shocked, they didn't show it. But it was true. During the past year, Bunny Boy had finally sprayed me, exhibiting a male bunny's ultimate sign of love and affection. I was now his soulmate.

"Biscuit keeps me fighting," said Jennifer, with a look that told me she understood my absolute love for Bunny Boy. "I wasn't blessed with any children."

Then Julie got it. She jumped into the conversation. "My dad says he wants to come back in his next life as a bunny. He thinks my mom sounds like a steamy romance novel when she talks to Bunny Boy."

I threw my arms around her, happy to share my life with a loving daughter who tolerated my boasting about Bunny Boy.

I was the last patient to leave the center that afternoon. My infusion had to be stopped for an hour midway, around noon, when my fever rose to 102 and my blood pressure was not within the acceptable range. When the nurse resumed the IV, the medication flowed more slowly to prevent that from happening again.

By the time we got home, I was extremely weak and nauseous. Ward had to help me walk into the house. Bunny Boy came sprinting across the kitchen and binkied so high when he saw me that I caught him in midair, surprising myself, wondering where I had found the strength. He had an amazing way of distracting and comforting me. From the look on Ward's and Julie's faces, they saw it as well.

Chapter 21

By Thanksgiving, I was feeling better. For the past few weeks, the warmth of Bunny Boy's furry body soothed my fever chills and eased the chest pain and nearly constant charley horses—muscle spasms—which were the side effects of my IV gamma globulin treatment. I was content—thankful for Bunny Boy's companionship.

I could barely contain my excitement as the mammoth-size Energizer Bunny strolled down Fifth Avenue on the TV. Bunny Boy and I snuggled happily under a blanket as we watched the Macy's Thanksgiving Day Parade together—a Buchalski childhood tradition that I tried to bring into our family. But as Julie and Chris got older, they lost interest and I was the only one who continued to watch the parade, so I was thrilled to have Bunny Boy's company.

I heard a commotion from the kitchen. Julie and Chris had found the *turkey* cake. It was my newest addition to the Thanksgiving menu. Julie's fluorescent tennis ball cake paled in comparison. The three-dimensional turkey chocolate cake was filled with chocolate ganache, and it sported orange, yellow, brown, and white buttercream feathers. Brilliantly, I thought it could double as both the centerpiece and dessert.

Chris had a great idea. "Bunny Boy's birthday is in December, Mom. Why haven't we made a bunny cake for him?" I was amazed I hadn't thought of it myself. My brow furrowed as I imagined all the critical missed opportunities for Bunny Boy's photo album.

When Bunny Boy spotted Chris, he dove off my lap and headed for Chris, bobbing like a boxer. He had had enough of the parade; it was time for some serious male bonding. Bunny Boy grabbed Chris's socks with his teeth and started thrashing his head back and forth like he was shaking a tattered doll. Then he lunged for Chris's ankles, as if he could tackle him. Chris dropped to the floor and they wrestled playfully on the rug until Bunny Boy rolled over on his back, looking for a belly rub.

"Mom, look! Bunny Boy's drooling."

I was so engrossed in the parade I hadn't noticed the saliva stain on my jeans. Drooling meant it was time to have Bunny Boy's molars trimmed again, which involved light anesthesia. The chewed moldings and gnawed shoes of Bunny Boy's earlier years now seemed desirable. Every two weeks, we drove up to Scuffy's, and Loretta would trim Bunny Boy's top and bottom front teeth. His molars were slower-growing and only needed to be trimmed every nine months.

"We'll schedule an appointment with Dr. Welch for Monday," I said. I still couldn't believe we had a bunny with as many health issues as I did. We were two peas in a pod.

During Thanksgiving dinner with the extended family, a crowd of twenty, no one could decide who or what was sillier—Bunny Boy or the cake. Or me, for that matter. I was a wild card—and so was Bunny Boy. When it came time for dessert, I couldn't bring myself to dismember the gorgeous display of turkey feathers in the middle of the table, so Bunny Boy did it for me. He popcorned from my lap, knocking over my glass and sending red wine pouring over the feathers, melting them and creating a pool of colorful mush. The cake was history.

Chris grabbed Bunny Boy and shook his paw. "I hated that cake, pal."

• • •

I had scheduled my second gamma globulin infusion for the day after Thanksgiving, thinking I would have Ward around for the long weekend to help out. But it suddenly registered in my brain that having eight hours of gamma globulin a day or two before such an important event as cutting down our Christmas trees might not have been a smart thing to do. But there wasn't a chance I would miss out on one of my favorite family traditions.

Every year for the last twenty years, my entire extended family would invade Black Oak Farms in Clinton, New Jersey, on Thanksgiving weekend. Rain or shine, no exceptions. Our caravan of cars would make the trip to western New Jersey to help thin out their pine tree inventory. The proprietor of the quaint farm lived on the property in an old, white shingled house with black shutters and a wraparound porch. Wild bunnies scurried through the fields. Over the years, we had seen an occasional coyote or fox, hence Bunny Boy had to skip the occasion.

When Ward expressed concern that I planned to go along so soon after my infusion, I reminded him of an old story. One year, I had asked Ward to make the hot chocolate for the trip while I packed some snacks. Unbeknownst to me, he boiled it. When a van swerved into our lane, the thermos, which was standing between my legs on the floor in the front seat, rolled to the right and the push-down top hit my knee. Boiled chocolate milk spilled into my boot, charring my ankle. Our line of family cars changed course and sped to the first emergency room along the route. The doctor cautiously removed my boot and peeled off my sock, which was stuck to the black, burnt skin on my ankle. I had a third-degree burn, but I had survived worse. There was no way I was going home that day without my Christmas trees.

It would be the same this year. "I guess we're going," Ward smiled.

But my second infusion, taken a day before, was proving difficult. The side effects of the treatments were cumulative, specifically the muscle cramping and fatigue. I tried to keep a stiff upper lip as I forced myself to climb the mountainous terrain in my weakened state, searching for two trees. Julie and Chris favored the weeping white pines with their long, pale-green needles. I preferred the Douglas firs with their soft, deep-green needles. Ward cut down one of each.

The following weekend, we put up the trees while snacking on a variety of appetizers and sipping hot chocolate spiked with peppermint schnapps. It was a circus, but it was *our* circus—strings of lights didn't work, ornaments broke, and a tray of food was flipped by our furry friend. It was safe to say that setting up the trees was Bunny Boy's favorite day of the year. He would grab the lights on the floor with his paws or teeth and roll over, tangled in the wires. Or he would pounce on the ornaments and drag them to the corner of the room.

When we finished, the weeping white pine stood in front of the picture window in the lagomorph lounge, adorned with brightly colored lights, silver beaded roping, giant Christmas plaid ribbon bows I had made, and the dozens of ornaments our family had collected over the years, which included hand-painted blown glass bunnies, wooden bunnies, bunnies made of hay, and a clear glass ornament with a photo of Bunny Boy inside, flanked by pictures of Julie and Chris. Ornaments of value were placed on the higher branches while ones that had seen better days were left at the bottom for Bunny Boy to have fun with. And he did—with ornaments to pillage, thick branches to burrow under, tinsel and pine needles that would get stuck to his paws, and a generous covering of branches to lounge under.

Then, under duress, Ward dragged the second tree into the sunroom. He strung it with lights, but nothing more. "One tree is plenty," he teased every year. But I disagreed and decorated the tree with the same enthusiasm as I did the first.

The tree in the sunroom was mine and Bunny Boy's. The shimmering lights were white and the ornaments were gold and cream. It had an elegance. Most nights, once everyone had gone to bed, Bunny Boy and I would hunker down on the sofa and just stare at the mystical, twinkling gift from nature. The hundreds of lights reflected off the glass windows that ran from the ceiling to the floor, and beams of light formed a starburst on the ceiling. I would relax and think about the many things I was grateful for. And I talked to Bunny Boy about everything. Sometimes, I complained about my health, too.

Later that night, Bunny Boy and I made our first nightly sojourn to the sunroom to enjoy our tree. I was decked in fleece bunny pajamas and larger-than-life bunny slippers that Ward had bought me for Valentine's Day. Suddenly, I tripped over the mammoth slippers and fell forward, sending Bunny Boy flying like a projectile across the room. He landed on the hard floor, nose first, missing the rug by only inches. He shook his head from side to side, then brought his front paws up to his mouth and scratched the area under his nose. I pried open his mouth. Two of his bottom front teeth were broken down to the gum line. Out of the corner of my eye, I spotted the shards of teeth on the floor.

"Are you okay, pal?" I asked, worried he might have injured his fragile jaw. He jerked his head away, which was uncharacteristic of him, but then he hopped up onto the sofa as if he was fine.

"I need to take one more look, Bunny Boy," I said firmly. He crouched down low and belly crawled to the end of the couch. Then he tore under the tree and hid. I peeked under.

"Are you okay, Bunny Boy?" I repeated.

A papier-mâché ornament came rolling toward me, and within seconds he was zigzagging under the tree with tinsel hanging from his broken teeth. "I guess you're fine, buddy," I said, before I headed up to bed. "I'll leave your teeth for the tooth fairy."

• • •

The next morning, Chris found Bunny Boy hunched over and sitting in a brown puddle in the spare bedroom. He was drooling unsightly liquid. His dewlap, nose, and front paws were drenched, and his body language told me he was tense. He stunk like bad garbage and thumped loudly several times. Gently, I tried to wipe his mouth with a warm washcloth but he jerked his head backward and took off across the room. His mouth was clearly hurting him. He thumped again, loudly, and started grinding his teeth. I called Dr. Welch immediately and set up an appointment.

The worst had happened.

Bunny Boy had broken his jaw in the exact spot where the surgeon had shaved off a piece of the bone. According to Dr. Welch, he would probably not survive the next forty-eight hours.

"That's impossible," I shrieked. "I'll force-feed him if I have to." I fought back tears. She had to be wrong. This couldn't possibly be happening to our bunny.

"Even if Bunny Boy can handle the pain, it will be nearly impossible to keep him inactive long enough for the jaw to heal," said Dr. Welch with a sense of urgency.

"I'll hold him all day if that's what it takes," I cried out.

"I will try to keep him comfortable," said Dr. Welch, choking on her words, reaching for my hand. "I'm so sorry, Mrs. Laracy. I know how much you love Bunny Boy. We all do."

She actually thought Bunny Boy was going to die. I was terrified.

While I never wanted Bunny Boy to suffer, I simply refused to accept the fact that he might die from a broken jaw. Bunny Boy was tough. I knew he was. Pain was no stranger to him—or me.

"I'll give Bunny Boy a shot for the pain and some liquid pain medication to take home with you," said Dr. Welch, kissing the top of Bunny Boy's head.

"Why the brown drool?" I managed to ask.

"Bunny Boy is eating his cecotropes and harboring them in his mouth until they're liquified."

While bunnies eat some of their cecotropes to keep their digestive track healthy, Bunny Boy was eating them as his primary food source. It was, and would be, too painful to eat his pellets.

I walked to the car clutching Bunny Boy, crying my eyes out. "You can't give up, Bunny Boy. I won't let you," I sobbed.

Bunny Boy looked up at me, listless and glazed. I sat in the front seat of the car and yelled out desperately. "There's no way I'll let you die from a broken jaw, buddy. You can beat this. I know you can."

I felt so helpless, so frightened. And I was rattled. How would I tell my family? I started praying with fervor until I could pull myself together enough to drive.

I pulled out of the parking lot with Bunny Boy resting on my lap, drooling onto my sweatpants. I must have still been partially dazed when I cut off a teenager in his souped-up jeep. He slammed on his horn, startling us. Bunny Boy plunged down onto my right foot and my car veered forward. My chest hit the steering wheel and I yanked the wheel toward the shoulder of the road while trying to lift my foot off the gas pedal, but Bunny Boy felt like an anvil. I managed to hit the brake with my left foot and threw the car into park. And then I screamed out of sheer frustration. My nerves had finally had enough.

"You nearly got us both killed, Bunny Boy," I shrieked amid my crying, as I lifted Bunny Boy off my foot. "Did you hear me buddy? What if I hadn't been able to control the car?" He stared at me with a glassy look, still in the land of psychedelic lights from his pain shot. Suddenly, he darted across the seat and looked around sharply, as if a danger was within striking distance, and started scratching wildly at the window. Then I saw the cop. I rolled down the window.

"He was sitting on my lap, officer, when a car horn scared him and he hopped onto the gas pedal. I think we're both fine." I was anything but fine. Bunny Boy was clawing madly at the front seat.

"We were just going home," I continued, reaching for a Kleenex to wipe away my tears. "It's been a rough time at the veterinarian."

The officer glanced at my drugged, psychotic bunny and kindly offered to follow me home, turning off his lights.

On the drive home, I decided I couldn't bear to tell my family about Bunny Boy's dismal prognosis. Instead, I focused on a plan for Bunny Boy's complete recovery. It was as simple as that.

"Bunny Boy has a broken jaw, but he is going to be fine," I told everyone as I kissed Ward's head gently, trying not to cry.

I gave Bunny Boy his pain medicine and fed him his critical care food around the clock like it was business as usual. He took them both compliantly. I rocked him for hours on end and slept with him on the bed in the spare room. I begged him not to give up. The tears dripped onto my T-shirt like icicles melting in the sun. I was frightened and completely heartbroken. It was gut-wrenching to watch Bunny Boy thump and grind his teeth, but my only consolation those first few days was when he would nudge me sweetly with the side of his face. I could still see some life in his eyes.

All plans for the holiday party we had offered to host for Ward's work had been put on hold. Each night, I said the rosary and begged God to help Bunny Boy recover. I couldn't imagine life without him. Ward told Julie and Chris the gravity of the situation, skipping the part that he could die. I asked the children to intensify their prayers and told them not to give me any presents for Christmas. Bunny Boy would be my gift if he lived, god willing.

By the fourth day after his accident, Bunny Boy had miraculously stopped grinding his teeth and thumping. He was still lethargic and showed no signs of wanting to be held by anyone except me. The kids and Ward took turns hanging out on the floor curled up next to him, stroking and talking to him. My family's love for Bunny Boy seemed to have deepened even further.

After a week of almost twenty-four-hour care, Bunny Boy was bobbing his head with a gentle enthusiasm for the apple banana goop. A brilliance returned to his eyes and his body seemed relaxed. Beneath my outer calm and positive facade, I still feared that his jaw might never heal properly. But that didn't matter for now. Bunny Boy had survived over two hundred and fifty hours, disregarding professional opinion. Dr. Welch was simply amazed.

"Bunny Boy has broken all rules when it comes to rabbits," she said. "He has the heart of a lion, not the prey animal he is. He is incredibly strong and tolerant of both pain and stress. As I've always said, the love and devotion from you and your family has made his heart stronger."

With each passing day, Bunny Boy regained his strength and light-heartedness. Our household slowly returned to some sense of normalcy, whatever normal was. By mid-December, I finally felt comfortable enough to leave Bunny Boy for more than an hour with Julie and Chris so I could attend a Christmas party with Ward. I called the caterer the next morning. Our holiday party was back on.

Chapter 22

By the time my birthday arrived on December 19, I had cut Bunny Boy's syringe feedings from four to twice a day. He was already eating the timothy hay pellets I had softened with warm water. He had also stopped drooling. His beautiful long ears, which had lain flat on his head for so long, returned to their "happy" position, and his nose resumed its twittering. According to Dr. Welch, Bunny Boy's recovery was a miracle and a testament to his incredible will to live.

But in true Laracy flip-flop style, my birthday turned into the night from hell. As we were about to turn in for the night, Chris ran into our bedroom clutching Sunny, showing us her stomach. There was a lump in our lizard's abdomen. Sunny looked like she was nine months pregnant.

"It wasn't there this morning," he shrieked. "We need to take her to the vet now!"

Speechless, I deferred to Ward. When he suggested we wait until morning, Chris practically convulsed and started crying. Ward mouthed quietly to me, "What's with our pets and lumps?"

"We have to take Sunny tonight, not tomorrow. It's huge, Mom."

Besides needing live crickets and worms, which required several trips a week to Scuffy's, Sunny had been a low-maintenance pet for seven years. She had never been to a vet, unlike Bunny Boy, a frequent flyer.

Ward took Chris to Oradell Animal Hospital, twenty-four-hour facility. He called home around midnight. Sunny either had an ovulated, unfertilized egg in her stomach that had not passed and had gotten infected—or she had a tumor. Neither scenario was good. The veterinarian suggested they leave her overnight for observation to the tune of several hundred dollars.

"Let me speak to your mother alone," I heard Ward say in the background. "Nance," he whispered. "Come on, it's a lot of money for a lizard, don't you think?"

"Of course it is, but it's Chris's pet," I said, thinking about the thousands of dollars we had spent on Bunny Boy. "If it were Bunny—"

He cut me off. "She's a lizard, Nance."

But I was firm, and he acquiesced. Sunny would stay overnight.

They returned after two in the morning. Chris crawled into bed with me while Ward slept in his room. Throughout the night, Chris called out Sunny's name several times in his sleep. It broke my heart. Sunny was Chris's first pet—a hand-me-down. When Julie had asked for an animal for Christmas one year, we ruled out dogs and cats because of Ward's allergies and hamsters and birds because of Julie's asthma. The tiny Australian bearded dragon hatchling arrived Christmas morning with a glass terrarium, a mound of supplies, and two plastic cups. One was full of crickets, the other full of mealworms. Julie looked at the creature in disbelief. "Whose idea was this? Chris's?" she said.

It didn't take more than a week or two of trying to toss live crickets and mealworms into the terrarium for Julie to pass down the lizard. Chris jumped right in and successfully raised Sunny from her pinky-finger size to a stately eighteen inches long. She was a healthy, pristine, well-trained reptile who hung out on a log beneath her sunlamp for hours and ate crickets, worms, and an abundance of leafy greens. She was also Bunny Boy's friend, sometimes taking rides on his back.

In the morning after his restless sleep, Chris's forehead felt hot.

"I think he's got a fever," I said when Ward came into the room.

I gave Chris some Tylenol and tucked him back under the covers. Bunny Boy appeared, hopping up onto the bed and burrowing under the blanket. Happily, I realized it was the first time he had hopped onto anything since he broke his jaw. As he snuggled into Chris's armpit, he started purring for the first time since his surgery. Our beloved Bunny Boy was back! We could always rely on him to comfort any one of us, at any given time. His instincts never failed him.

It was the day of the holiday party. I had to get everything ready—but there was also the matter of Sunny. I went into party mode, washing glassware, folding red and green napkins, and baking about eight dozen cookies. Then I called the veterinarian. Sadly, Sunny had cancer, and the veterinarian said she could be suffering. We would have to euthanize her.

I walked upstairs to break my little boy's heart.

"I want to speak to the veterinarian," Chris said, trying to push back his emotion. With great courage, his voice cracking, Chris asked the doctor, "Is putting Sunny to sleep my only choice?"

I watched as Chris listened to the other end of the line. Then he said, "I can't watch her suffer. I love her too much." Tears trickled down his warm cheeks. "I'll pick Sunny up this afternoon," he said, as if he'd be driving to the vet himself. Then he hung up.

I brought my sick, heartbroken little boy back to bed, twirling his soft hair between my fingers until he fell back to sleep. I was feeling choked up myself, and also overwhelmed. We had fifty guests coming around six o'clock, and we had to end the life of one of our family pets.

I called the animal hospital back. "Is it possible to pick Sunny up tomorrow?" I asked. There was a ghastly sigh at the end of the receiver. I capitulated.

I assigned the task of picking up Sunny's remains to Ward and resumed my party preparations. My body pain was escalating rapidly from the stress and sheer physical work but I refused to give in and pushed myself, sitting down in between tasks and focusing on the goal at hand, while also handling a burst pipe in the basement and checking on Chris, Julie, and the caterers, who had just arrived. When Bunny Boy met them enthusiastically at the front door, one of the caterers backed up, frightened, thinking he was a baby fox, while the other tripped, nearly dropping a platter of cocktail sandwiches. The third stepped over him as though he were a stuffed animal left on the floor by a child.

Then I got ready, stepping into the shower and turning the water onto the hottest setting I could handle to soak my pain-ridden body. I literally began to laugh. What else could I do? We were a nuthouse. I dried off and put a lidocaine patch on my lower back to ease the muscle pain. The six-by-eight-inch patches, which had recently become available through prescription by my doctor, were invaluable for small areas, and I had to keep them on for twelve hours. Then I stepped into my black velvet dress with matching pumps and curled my hair loosely with electric curlers; blow-drying my hair was too difficult for my sore arms. "You clean up well," said one of the caterers. I wasn't sure whether to be complimented or offended.

When Ward came in, he was carrying a small pink box.

"Is that Sunny?" I asked somberly, reaching to kiss him in gratitude.

"No, it's a late birthday present for you. Of course, it's her."

My eyes welled up. "Let's call Chris down to see her. Sadly, we will have to put her in the freezer." I felt pained and heartless, but we didn't have time for a proper burial.

"May I take that?" One of the caterers had just walked in. "Do you have a small platter I can put the chocolates on?" she asked, gesturing to the pink box.

"It's our dead lizard," I said in a deadpan tone. "Not chocolates."

She looked at me as if she could not have possibly heard me right.

Chris turned the corner into the kitchen, sporting a crisp pair of black pants, a white shirt, and a Christmas plaid bowtie. He still insisted that he was in charge of pouring the champagne for our guests. He looked dashing except for his glassy eyes. Ward handed him the pink box.

"I tried to take such good care of her," he said. I sensed a gush of tears was imminent.

Chris carried Sunny up to the playroom and sat on the sofa, fiddling with the pink box and talking to her. When Bunny Boy approached and swatted the package with his front paws, Chris lost his temper with our bunny for the first time since Bunny Boy shredded his Nintendo wires. Bunny Boy scampered away, his ears flat. He knew he had done something to upset Chris. I picked him up and put on his Santa hat.

By the time the holiday guests arrived, Sunny was tucked away safely in the freezer in the garage, and soon many of our guests were taking turns holding our Christmas bunny, feigning their love for rabbits.

• • •

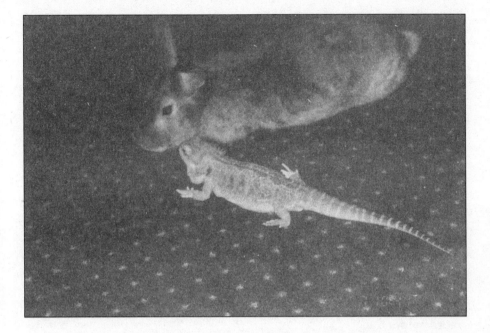

On the morning of Christmas Eve, we had yet to bury Sunny. She was still nestled among the Buffalo chicken strips and Skinny Cow ice cream sandwiches. Twelve inches of snow had fallen the day after our holiday party, but Chris was adamant.

"I want to bury Sunny today."

Of course, he had chosen to bury our lizard on one of the busiest days of the year. Christmas Eve was the most important holiday celebration for the Buchalskis. Our tradition stemmed back to the year my father died in 1981. That year, we had gathered at my childhood home on December 24, just nineteen days after Dad had left us. We mourned our profound loss together, but amid our sadness, we stumbled upon something. Being together on Christmas Eve left Christmas Day free for my brothers to spend the holiday with their in-laws. So began our family tradition of celebrating on Christmas Eve, which the Laracys have been hosting since Ward and I were married.

With so much preparation to do before my family arrived, I felt myself going into Martha mode, but then I stopped. I forced myself to become Mary for a moment. How meaningful would it be to bury Sunny on Christmas Eve? After all, she had come to us one special Christmas Day.

"I think that's a fantastic idea, Chris," I said, kissing the top of his head.

I went to the tree to fetch a silver gift box addressed to Chris. It contained Sunny's headstone. I had picked it up from our local garden center and had planned on giving it to Chris on Christmas morning. I slipped it into my pocket and then went to retrieve Sunny. Chris's lip quivered when he saw the pink box. He started rummaging through the kitchen cabinets and closets, desperately looking for an airtight container for Sunny. He feared the insects would get to her once she was buried. I had an idea. I opened the refrigerator and took out my two Christmas tins packed full of baked goods that I had been making all week. I arranged half of the brownies and cookies on a platter and consolidated the rest in another container.

"We can put Sunny is this."

"Sunny came to us on Christmas, and now she's leaving us on Christmas Eve in a Christmas tin." He beamed. "It's perfect."

Within minutes, our funeral procession moved slowly across the yard. Underneath our winter coats, the kids and I were still in our Christmas jammies; Ward had on Christmas boxer shorts. Julie and I squeezed together under my umbrella as a gentle rain fell, leaving tiny holes in the melting snow. Bunny Boy was cradled in Julie's arms. Chris led us deep into the woods. I thought of Flop, picturing our family's funeral procession of seven and her grave in the backyard of my childhood home.

Chris chose a spot in a small clearing behind a holly bush. Ward dug a hole as I said a few prayers. Then, I pulled out the silver box from my pocket.

"What's this, Mom?" Chris asked.

"Open it and see."

Chris gingerly unwrapped the box with his small hands.

"Oh, Mom and Dad, it's perfect."

We were ready. Ward placed the Christmas tin in the hole and covered it with dirt. The sound of the soft raindrops on the bushes and the rustling of the squirrels provided a beautiful, natural background chorus while we said our tearful goodbye to Sunny, huddled together in the woods on Christmas Eve.

When we returned to the house, Julie put Bunny Boy down, and he darted across the family room and stopped short in front of Sunny's terrarium. He stared through the glass, like he had done for the past few days. Then he stood up on his hind legs, stretched his head down into the glass container, and sniffed around, clearly looking for her.

I had forgotten that Bunny Boy was in mourning, too.

By noon, exhausted from all the gift wrapping and holiday preparations, I took my usual cocktail of four Advil tablets and Tylenol and curled up to rest on the sofa with my version of Red Bull—two Earl Grey tea bags steeping in my Santa mug. Recharged, I got up and found Julie and Chris in the kitchen—equally recharged from chocolate and sugar! They had skipped right over lunch and were popping my holiday cookies into their mouths. The platter was looking sparse, so I reached for the remaining Christmas tin, hoping to replenish the platter—

"Waaaaaaaard!" I screamed, racing toward the landing to the stairs. "She's here! Sunny's here!"

There was Sunny's pink box, in the tin. We had mixed the boxes!

We all hovered over the tin, staring in disbelief.

"So, let me get this straight, Nance. You're telling me that I buried the desserts?" Ward said.

Our nuthouse had just gotten nuttier.

• • •

Besides our little mishap, Christmas was as wonderful and joyous as it always was. Despite the amount of pain it caused me to decorate the house and host parties, I was determined to push through to create the perfect "Bing Crosby Christmas." Our lawn was lit up with two reindeer constructed of wood and wire, and a giant, spotlighted wreath with a red velvet bow hung on our door. Fresh wreaths hung on the six ground-floor windows, and artificial candles lit up the windows on the second floor. Whenever we returned to the house and approached the porch, we would see Bunny Boy through the window, sitting on his haunches and gazing up at the twinkling lights. He looked absolutely enchanting, like a Norman Rockwell image. Inside, the living room was decked out in gold, the perfect backdrop for fresh pine wreathing, antique-style felt fruit clusters, white poinsettias, and large gold bows. Dozens of white votives scattered among the tables gave the room a soft glow, and brass sconces wrapped in fresh mistletoe flanked the mantel. The wooden stairway leading up to the landing was draped with wreaths, magnolia leaves, mistletoe, white pine swags, and over-sized plaid bows. Bunny Boy was often found swatting the greenery on the railings with his forceful back paws when he got bored with the Christmas trees.

It was my Christmas wonderland.

Christmas was special for a few other reasons that year. Bunny Boy had beaten the odds and was still very much alive. Ward had also found my favorite gold bracelet that I thought I had lost forever at one of his corporate parties, on the mat of the passenger seat in the car. It was seemingly impossible.

"Someone wanted to make sure you had a Christmas present other than Bunny Boy," Ward said, shaking his head in disbelief. I felt as if an angel had wrapped its wings around me.

That Christmas night, Bunny Boy took his very first swim in the hot tub. The whole family had gathered in the outdoor jacuzzi, and Chris had plopped Bunny Boy onto the deck in the snow. He popcorned bliss-fully, sending powder flying into the air and leaving paw prints across the snow-covered deck. Then, he fell on his side and started wiggling his back paws, forming his own snow angel. His face was sprinkled with snow, making him look like a sugared confection. Bunny Boy was in snow bunny heaven.

Soon, Bunny Boy was as intrigued with the hot tub as he was with the snow, and he took his place among our family soak—accidentally. He binkied too close to the edge, falling in butt-first. Bunny Boy started tun-neling and swimming like an otter, frantically, swallowing some water.

"Grab him!" I screamed, jumping from my seat.

His wet, thrashing body slipped through our hands. Bunny Boy was in survival mode, oblivious to all of us. But Julie, with her calm and cool demeanor, came to Bunny Boy's rescue. She grabbed her towel from the railing and scooped him up.

"You're a lunatic, Bunny Boy!" I shrieked, sounding like a lunatic myself, fearing that the exposure to the bitter cold and the 104-degree water might cause him to have a heart attack.

We traipsed into the sunroom, tracking snow all over the rug. Bunny Boy's soggy, wet head stuck out of the towel as he licked himself profusely. He seemed no worse for the wear. His nose was twittering at the appropriate speed and his ears were straight up in the "happy" position—my bunny vital signs.

"You gotta love Bunny Boy, Nance," said Ward. "He doesn't want to miss a thing."

"Spa night's over for everyone," I said. "Except Bunny Boy. Julie and I will blow-dry him upstairs."

Ward closed up the hot tub. It was twelve fifteen. Our magical Christmas was over.

Chapter 23

Another New Year's came and went. Bunny Boy's jaw healed perfectly against all odds, and by mid-March my gamma globulin infusions were finished. With great trepidation but little choice, I had started giving myself injections of Enbrel. The parvovirus antibodies had been suppressed by the gamma globulin treatment, and now the Enbrel would hopefully treat the connective tissue disease in the long term. Sadly, my usual short protocols of the steroid prednisone were no longer keeping my connective tissue disease under control. Steroids are extremely effective for short-term use, but when used over many years in the long term, they are dangerous and can shut down your entire immune system instead of just one part of it. Now that I was on Enbrel, I was feeling stronger and more energetic than I had in a long time.

It was time for spring cleaning.

I compiled a list of jobs to be done in the upcoming weeks and delegated like a true corporate executive. Julie and Chris protested the event vehemently, as they did each year and as I had when I was younger. Tina, the dear that she was, went into overdrive, ticking off items on the list I had posted on the refrigerator. Closets and cabinets were reorganized and thinned out. Bags of trash and old clothes, school supplies, and toys, along with dozens of magazines and books, were piled up in the garage like the Grinch had come through. "It's gotta go," Tina said. Meanwhile, I was just in drive, and Julie and Chris were parked. On the sofa next to Bunny Boy.

When I returned home one afternoon, I noticed that the door to the lagomorph lounge was only open a crack. Hoping to sneak up on Bunny

Boy and give him a big smooch, I opened the door slowly. I broke into hilarious laughter when I saw Bunny Boy on the carpet, sloshing around in white frothy foam with the distinct smell of lavender. He seemed to be enjoying a good bubble bath. But I was also puzzled.

It turned out that Tina had sprayed deodorized carpet shampoo on the rug. She thought she had closed the door, but our nosey, mischievous bunny must have squeezed through the small opening. Tina had found the can of carpet cleaner in the garage; it had to be at least six years old, pre–Bunny Boy. The label read "pet-safe," but I didn't trust it. I gave Bunny Boy a real bath in the kitchen sink while Tina vacuumed up the foam. Then we closed off the room securely until the rug could dry.

After his bath, Bunny Boy stationed himself on the landing to the family room and looked up at me, waiting for me to open the door.

"It's off limits, Bunny Boy!" I said sternly.

He stood on his hind legs and started scratching at the door. He sniffed the gap between the floor and the door, then flipped his hind legs forcefully against the door, trying to open it. I was amazed at the strength of his thumper legs and the loud sound they made. I ignored him, and my lack of concern for his plight seemed to anger him. He tore down the stairs after me, leaving caution to the wind and grabbing my pants with his teeth, trying to get me to follow him up to the landing.

"You have full run of this house, Bunny Boy. Choose another room for the time being." I playfully grabbed his fluffy tail. I got nowhere.

Bunny Boy had no interest in hanging out in any other rooms. The lagomorph lounge was his fortress. He pounded the door a second time with his hind legs, startling both of us. He finally gave up and laid against the door, downtrodden.

"The room's fair game in the morning, Bunny Boy."

That night, I bribed him off the landing with a piece of banana and brought him to our bed. He swallowed the banana slice whole but refused my apology and dove onto Ward's side of the bed defiantly.

I slipped under the covers, foraged around for my rosary beads, and started to pray, acting as if I couldn't care less that Bunny Boy had snubbed me. Bunny Boy rolled over playfully on Ward's lap and looked my way, hoping to get my attention. So I kept praying. He tugged at the string on Ward's pajama pants and binkied to the bottom of the bed. He thumped the thick down comforter and stared at me, desperately trying to get my attention.

"Our Father, who art in—" I started but never got any further. Bunny Boy lunged onto my lap and snatched the rosary beads, attacking them. Within moments, the crucifix was hanging from his teeth and the beads were tangled around his neck and front paws.

"Surrender the beads, Bunny Boy," I ordered jokingly. He started shaking the cross, causing the beads to tighten.

"The beads please, Bunny Boy?" I asked quietly, fearing his excitement might cause the beads to tighten around his fragile neck. Slowly, he put his front paws forward and his head down into the submissive position, admitting defeat and seeking my assistance.

Ever so slowly and skillfully, Ward and I unwrapped the beads. Almost in gratitude, Bunny Boy nestled on my chest and purred.

When I woke up the next morning, Bunny Boy was sitting on the landing, waiting again to be let in. I wondered if he had been there all night. I walked down the stairs slowly, taunting him.

"Good morning, Bunny Boy. How long have you been sitting there, pal?"

Bunny Boy started scratching at the door with a frenetic pace.

"Do you want to go back in your room?"

Bunny Boy flipped his hind legs and sprayed me.

"Bunny Boy just adores you, Nance," said Ward, who was watching from above.

"I know he does," I replied, rolling up the bottom of my pajama pants as if getting sprayed with urine was typical when you have a house rabbit who loves you. I opened the door and Bunny Boy tore across the room and sprung onto the sofa, scaling the back like a skilled rock climber. He plunged off the back headfirst, down into Julie's laundry basket, which was full of her old, overpriced Beanie Babies, and sent them sailing across the floor with his back legs. Bunny Boy was in his glory, back on his protected turf.

That day, my mother and I ventured out to buy spring flowers from Jake's Place, our local garden center that doubled up as a pet store. With some guilt, we left Bunny Boy at home as there was no room in the car. Bunny Boy loved visiting Jake's Place for its maze of corners and crevices he could explore, as well as for its namesake Jake, the store's large, gentle resident golden retriever who tolerated Bunny Boy's nosiness—and I knew he would be upset. When we returned home, Bunny Boy was waiting in the foyer, displaying some major bunny attitude with his body language. He hopped past me deliberately and sniffed my mother's feet, looking up at her in adoration.

"How's my favorite grandson?" Mom said. Bunny Boy gamboled into the kitchen, stopping to look back at her, hoping she would follow. I chased after him, trying to make amends, when I stumbled upon a mess. Bunny Boy's litter pan was flipped upside down and the contents were scattered all over. He flipped his hind legs up and plopped down on his side, looking at me as if to say, "Here's why you shouldn't have left me home."

"Come here, you silly old rabbit." I whisked him up, my arms aching from lugging all those flowers around. When I rolled Bunny Boy over to give him a big raspberry on his belly, I gasped. His underside was bright red and shiny, like a newly polished sports car—and it was full of scratch marks. Bunny Boy's beautiful white fur was gone. We ran up to the family room and found clumps of fur scattered around the freshly cleaned carpet.

"He was a very busy rabbit while we were out," Mom said. "And he clearly had an allergic reaction to the carpet cleaner. You better get him to the vet."

Bunny Boy spent the car ride over to Franklin Lakes Animal Hospital licking himself, irritating his skin even more. Sheri, one of the technicians we had come to know, was standing behind the front desk when we barged in.

"And why is Bunny Boy here today, Mrs. Laracy?" she asked, referencing the fact that we came to visit more often than most pets did.

"He ripped out the fur on his chest. I believe he had a bad reaction to some carpet cleaner."

She looked at me, aghast.

"This is relatively minor," said Dr. Welch once she examined him. "Bunny Boy's one tough rabbit. I'll give him a shot of steroids to stop the allergic reaction and some cream to put on his stomach."

I felt worn out. I thought back to his broken jaw, which hadn't been his fault, much like the carpet cleaner.

"There's no charge for this one," Dr. Welch said. "Try to relax, Mrs. Laracy."

Bunny Boy was hyper for the rest of the day. I should have recognized the familiar signs. On the ride home, he circled the seat of the car like a dog chasing its tail, hopping from the seat to the floor and back up again. At the house, Bunny Boy dove out of my arms and started racing around, skidding into everything, darted from one piece of furniture to the next, sniffing the wood, licking the fabric, and pawing wildly. Julie and Chris egged him on, chasing him around and wrestling him on the carpet until he should have collapsed from exhaustion. But Bunny Boy didn't let up.

I tried to start dinner, but the fun and chaos from the living room drew me back in. When I walked through the archway leading into the room, I saw Bunny Boy fly at least eight feet from the sofa across the living room, as if he had been shot out of a canon. He was panting heavily, and his nose was twittering faster than I had ever seen. His whiskers flapped wildly. His eyes looked like they might bulge right out of his head. Bunny Boy looked possessed.

"We have a jacked-up rabbit!" I yelled to the kids, once it dawned on me. "Dr. Welch gave Bunny Boy a shot of steroids."

Julie and Chris looked at each other, then at Bunny Boy, then at me. They knew what they were witnessing. They had seen me when I was on steroids. Dirty laundry that was left on the floor was thrown out the back door. Bedrooms got torn apart. Backpacks flew. Homework was marked up and sent back for revisions. Shoes got polished. Food that wasn't clearly marked became my property.

I, too, had been accused of looking possessed.

On top of the sofa, Bunny Boy pounced back and forth as if he was mirroring the movements of a pacing tiger. He looked at the hardwood floors on one side and the carpet on the other, weighing his choices.

"We need to get him down before he jumps," I said, as if we were luring him down from committing suicide. Finally, we cornered him and Bunny Boy leapt onto Chris's shoulder, balancing there on his haunches like a parrot.

"Calm down, little man," Chris whispered, gently petting his head.

"You're going to be fine, sweetie," said Julie, rubbing noses with him.

I wished I had a camera and a tape recorder nearby. When *I* went on a steroid rage, I never heard those words; instead, I heard hostile voices: "Calm down, Mom. You're acting insane!"

But Bunny Boy was incapable of calming down. He flew off the chair and crashed dangerously into the coffee table. Then he leapt up to the back of the sofa again, skipping the seat.

I quickly called Dr. Welch.

"Just keep Bunny Boy safe. The drugs should wear off by morning."

"Safe? How?"

We removed the table and chairs from the kitchen and closed off the doorways with old baby gates. I camped out with Bunny Boy for the night. We were getting good at that.

At least for the next few hours, the bunny show was great.

Chapter 24

I had always enjoyed warm weather, even before my health challenges, but for a short while, it became my nemesis. I was sweating almost constantly for weeks on end, an anomaly for me; I typically only got the sweats when I experienced an adrenaline rush from a stressful trigger or when I was sick or had a flare up.

I was also sleeping less than usual. My energy had plummeted like Wall Street during a bear market. Sweaty sheets and laundry piled up, and many a night was spent hanging out with Bunny Boy watching chick flicks. He didn't seem to mind the fact that I was exceptionally irritable.

My annual checkup shed some light on the matter. I was in full-blown menopause. I had chalked up the heart palpitations and adrenaline rushes to raising two teens and Bunny Boy's antics. The loss of my monthly cycle, I assumed, was from the gamma globulin infusions. It had happened once before, though temporarily. It had never occurred to me that the Enbrel injections I had started using this past winter could have been the culprit. Basically, my body had been shocked into menopause. I had had a five-year loss of estrogen in less than six months.

"Premature menopause can be quite debilitating," said my ob-gyn, Dr. Nicosia. "I'm surprised I didn't hear from you sooner, Nance."

While I was going through some significant changes, everyone else was growing up or growing old. Chris was in eighth grade, juggling a difficult course load, playing on two basketball teams, and still finding time for the video game Halo, which we had stood in line at midnight to purchase. Bunny Boy would pace back and forth on the sofa as Chris played, enjoying the graphics. Chris also arranged poker games for his friends, using the new table top I had lugged home from the mall, causing me to throw my back out. There was nothing I wouldn't do for my children.

The third season of spectacular girls' tennis had wrapped up, and as a high school junior, Julie won All State, All League, and All County. She had also fought competitively on the debate team, bringing home the school's first team trophy. In between her activities, we had also started looking at colleges.

My mother was approaching eighty years old. Her degenerative arthritis in her back and hip pains were slowing her down. She drove less and rested more, but rarely complained. Ward would turn fifty in the fall, though he didn't look a day over thirty-five. Daily workouts and healthy eating for most of his adult life had paid off.

And Bunny Boy was over five years old—geriatric, according to most sources I had read. The changes in his fur were more pronounced. Strands of brown were strewn throughout the base ginger color, as if he had a reverse highlighting. The fur on his belly was sparse. He moved at a slower pace and used more caution when hopping on and off furniture. His trips up to the bedrooms became less frequent. I tried to convince myself that he was being more careful due to his broken jaw, but who was I kidding?

When I clapped my hands to ignite the bunny game, Bunny Boy tore around with the same sparkle in his eyes, but with less gas. He also just hung out for a larger portion of the day, though he kept his crepuscular routine in the evening, settling in the lagomorph lounge around dusk with his toys and human playmates. Once Ward walked over at ten o'clock sharp to say "Goodnight, Bunny Boy," he knew I would be headed up to bed within the hour. He would binky over to wherever I was sitting and use any tactic to keep me from going to bed—tugging at my socks or pants until I chased him around or nudging his wicker ball in my path playfully, nearly tripping me. Ultimately, we would end up nesting on the recliner. I would whisper, "I love you more than life itself, Bunny Boy," or "What would I do without you, little buddy?" It was so easy to express my deepest feelings to him. We would rub noses or he would lick my cheeks and earlobes tenderly.

When I would finally start up the stairs to bed, Bunny Boy would sit on the landing and thump, demanding me to come back. Most times I did. If only for a short while.

• • •

"California is definitely out of the question." I said emphatically. "It's too far."

With Bunny Boy strategically tucked in my arms, I handed Julie a list of top-notch colleges I had compiled that were within three hours' driving distance of Bunny Boy. We all used him as a pawn at one time or another.

We had begun narrowing down college choices for Julie, and one of her criteria was warm weather all year round, not just in the summer. I raised the issue of college being situated close to Bunny Boy, but, really, I was also focused on Julie being close to me!

During spring break, we visited eight southern schools on the East coast due to their temperate weather and the fact that all of them were less than a ten-hour drive away. Though I dreaded the long hours in the car, which I knew would dramatically affect my pain for the worse, the trip ended up being some of the best family bonding time for us in a long while. We played games and sang silly songs—Julie put on her deep guttural voice as she pumped out tunes, in stark contrast to the candy-coated voice she used whenever she sang to Bunny Boy. We also vigorously discussed virtually every topic under the sun, including the upcoming 2008 election, where a female and black candidate were fighting for the top seat as the president of the United States. During our time away, Kelly, one of the technicians from Franklin Lakes Animal Hospital, made house calls to give Bunny Boy penicillin shots and bandage changes for a new, small abscess on one of his hocks. I called Kelly at the same time every day to check on him. She usually sounded out of breath when she answered the phone. Despite his geriatric status, Bunny Boy would make a mad dash for one of his many cozy spots in the house whenever Kelly showed up, reluctant to receive his shot from someone other than Ward. She tried bringing along her two toddlers to lure him out, with little success. It became a game of cat and mouse.

As we walked the sprawling lawns, quads, and bluestone walkways lined with magnolias and cherry blossoms while the sun shown overhead and the temperatures hovered in the seventies, it didn't take me long to decide I wanted to go to graduate school in the south—with Julie! As she and I skipped, arm in arm, I reminded her of the time she was in kindergarten when I told her a bedtime story about the Care Bears going off to college—to help her fall asleep.

"Can you be my class mother when I go to college?" she had asked with childhood innocence. That cherished moment was as clear to me as if it had been yesterday.

• • •

Wake Forest University was the final stop on our southern expedition. Its folder, containing the materials from the admissions department, had a picture of Bunny Boy taped to the front and a large red circle with a line drawn diagonally across it. In other words, *don't go here*. Geographically, it was the furthest school from home. I thought I was being subtle. Wake Forest was also the most academically challenging and conservative school on Julie's list. Right-wing views were the norm, politically and socially. I knew it was not a good match for Julie, our screaming liberal. Living just outside of Manhattan, our geographic area lent itself toward left-wing politics and morals. Our children were very open-minded when it came to issues like race, nationality, and religion, a value we instilled in them from an early age.

The morning of the Wake Forest tour, Julie walked out of the bathroom, almost unrecognizable. Her long, flowing brown hair was pulled back tight in a clip, and faux pearls replaced her Betsy Johnson dangling spider earrings. She was wearing khaki shorts and a light blue Lacoste collared shirt instead of jean shorts and a T-shirt with a witty slogan, her usual attire.

"It's my Wake Forest outfit," she announced. "I borrowed it from Amanda."

She looked lovely. Her conservative attire sat perfectly with me.

We walked the stunning Wake Forest campus. The girls wore Lily Pulitzer sundresses and strappy sandals with designer bags slung across their shoulders, while the men wore chino pants or shorts, collared golf shirts, and Docksiders. They looked like an advertisement for J. Crew. The campus was crawling with rich Caucasian kids, exactly what Julie was trying to escape. Chris put it simply: "If you need to borrow clothes to go here, Jules, it's not the school for you."

The sneeze cemented the thought. We were trailing behind our group, listening to the flawless, enthusiastic presentation of Miss Wake Forest Ra Ra, former prom queen, senior class president, and Most Likely to Succeed, when Ward sneezed. A Laracy sneeze could run a turbine or give someone a heart attack. The first time baby Julie sneezed, she nearly rolled off her changing table. That is a fact.

Our tour group spun around and glared at us with great disdain. You would have thought Ward had said he wanted to burn the American Flag. Julie ducked behind me, trying to hide. Ward went one step further.

"What can I say—if I hold in my sneeze, my head explodes," he declared.

I bent over laughing. Chris gave Ward a high five. Julie was so appalled she ran from our group and never looked back. We fled the campus, returning to the north where we belonged.

By the time we crossed the border into Pennsylvania, seven hours later, it was forty-one degrees outside and raining. Julie woke up from her nap and touched the ice-cold car window.

"I'm definitely going south for college, guys." Could I blame her?

We returned, tired and a little edgy. Bunny Boy was waiting at the top of the stairs when we walked in. He kicked his hind legs into the air playfully and took turns sniffing everyone's feet. There was a note on the counter from Kelly welcoming us back, signed with a happy face.

• • •

For the rest of the spring, we changed the bandage on Bunny Boy's paw daily, using bandages in bright spring colors—light pink, yellow, lavender, and mint green. Ward gave Bunny Boy his penicillin shots. And every time the sky had a hint of gray, rain fell, or the temperature dipped into the fifties, Julie gave me the latest weather report for the south.

Thankfully, summertime in the northeast quickly brought warmer temperatures and sunny skies. Our native rhododendrons were in full-bloom, some reaching up to ten feet tall, and the bright orange tulips had withered, making room for my favorite annuals, impatiens. Over the years, during these warm summer days, I often sat on the porch with Bunny Boy, which became a familiar sight in my neighborhood. Our neighbor Leslie, a die-hard walker and admirer of my flowers, would stroll across the lawn in her sweatpants and Keds sneakers to chat with me about Bunny Boy.

"I tell everybody about this bunny," she would say over and over again.

"He's my inspiration to keep fighting, Leslie," I would reply.

That summer, Julie and Chris were helping me to plan the ultimate fiftieth birthday surprise for Ward. He would hit the milestone, god willing, in November.

Napa Valley, California, was the obvious choice. Ward had been collecting wine since the late 1970s, and we had yet to travel to any vineyards outside of New Jersey. I made plans for us to arrive in San Francisco the day before his actual birthday and drive out to wine country the morning of the big day. I was so genuinely excited I thought I could burst.

By late October, nobody had leaked a word about the surprise trip. Chris, in particular, got my special praise. He and Ward were attached at the hip these days. They watched sci-fi movies into the wee hours of the morning. They jogged together. They lifted weights and practically lived on protein shakes. I could feel Chris drifting from me, normal for any teenage boy, but I sorely missed snuggling with him on the recliner and watching *Family Guy* or spending late afternoons at the Guitar Center embracing his new hobby and learning everything I could about guitars. My little buddy was not so little anymore.

In an effort to placate her parents, Julie had also reluctantly agreed to tour the College of New Jersey shortly before Ward and I had left for Napa Valley. Ward's brother and sister-in-law were adjunct professors at the very popular, highly competitive state school. After walking the campus for less than an hour, our screaming liberal daughter said, "The student body is so diverse. The kids seem just like me."

And she was right. There university was known for its liberal policies and political culture, and the campus exuded a comfortable casualness. The school had Division I sports if Julie wanted to play tennis and a strong academic program. Bunny Boy would also be only an hour and a half away.

Meanwhile, Bunny Boy was spending more and more of his time just hanging out in the lagomorph lounge. He had slowed down noticeably over the past few months. He was also leaving occasional poop pellets around the perimeter of his litter pan and along the bottom of the sofas. According to Dr. Welch, this was normal behavior with a geriatric bunny. She thought he might also be developing some arthritis. Although Bunny Boy was clearly aging, he was still strong and determined. None of his trials or tribulations had dulled his spirit. But the reality began to sink in with me.

Bunny Boy was my rock. He went about life with a joie de vivre that inspired me. He had lived over six years from the date of his first surgery and had survived numerous medical catastrophes. With each subsequent mishap or health issue, my prayers intensified. I asked God to keep Bunny Boy safe when he underwent anesthesia and prayed he would never die of a heart attack from pain. Most of all, I hoped I would never have to euthanize Bunny Boy. I wanted him to die in my arms one day.

A week before Ward's big surprise, Chris handed Ward a velvet wine bag containing the trip itinerary and two wine bottle Christmas ornaments. Bunny Boy was cradled in Julie's arms. I lit a Merlot-scented candle.

"Surpriiiiiiise!" we screamed in unison, startling Bunny Boy who lunged headfirst onto the glass coffee table and slid off the side. He scrambled onto all fours and thumped loudly. *Dear god, not another accident!* I thought. I shamefully blew Ward off to check on Bunny Boy.

"I want to come back in my next life as that rabbit," Ward remarked. "How about you kids?"

Bunny Boy's theatrics turned out to be nothing more than a scare, and our much-awaited trip to the wine country was everything I had hoped it would be—relaxing, rejuvenating, and romantic. When we returned, well-rested, we were ready to host Thanksgiving once again. Bunny Boy went solo on our Christmas card that year, perched in front of the tree with his Santa hat. He looked like an oversized beanie baby. It was one of his finer moments.

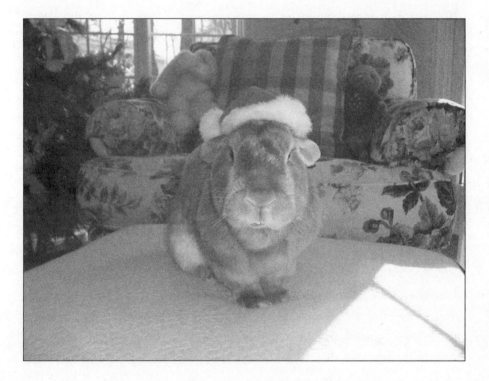

Chapter 25

By early February, the northeast had gotten pounded with eleven snow-
storms. It was already the snowiest winter on record since the 1940s.
It seemed Julie and Chris were home more than they were in school.
Even Bunny Boy had temporarily given up his recent couch potato status,
frolicking back and forth along the French doors in the sunroom chasing
snowflakes or pawing wildly at the glass doors as the kids slid down the
backyard on their snow tubes. I was ecstatic to see his renewed burst of
energy, and the thoughts of Bunny Boy aging were pushed to the back of
my mind, replaced by youthful images of my furry friend—the irresistible kit finding his way into our rambunctious family, the science projects
and sports games where he became the star, the many calamities or antics
that rendered us helpless as we laughed uncontrollably.

In February, we took a vacation to Puerto Rico. At first, getting
there looked like a crapshoot. Three out of the four of us had gotten the
dreaded stomach flu, though so far I had dodged the bullet, walking
around wearing a mask and carrying the Kaopectate and Lysol. But our
plans forged ahead, and we arranged for Kelly to drop by again to check
on Bunny Boy. Another small abscess had cropped up on the surface of
his face, and thankfully, we had caught it early.

The first wave of nausea hit me on the plane. The second came while
we waited at Julie's aptly named "baggage clam." By the time we reached
our hotel, I had vicious contents coming out from both ends of my anatomy. I quickly went into seclusion. I missed Bunny Boy. I wanted my
security blanket. But the stomach flu took its normal course, thankfully,
without causing any further complications. A few years back, during one

of our previous trips to Puerto Rico, chest pain and severe sweating and anxiousness, side effects from Celebrex, had sent me to the emergency room in the small town of Dorado. The antiquated EKG equipment consisted of four metal cuffs for my ankles and wrists that were attached to a small monitor. I sat there feeling I was about to be executed. Fortunately, it was a temporary issue, and I was able to stay on for the vacation.

Similarly, this time I recovered from the stomach flu soon enough to enjoy the warm weather, a perfect winter interlude for the whole family. On our return, there was a note on the counter from Kelly.

"Everything went fine, but call me when you have a minute." As I suspected, Kelly, too, had noticed that Bunny Boy was slowing down.

During this time, Chris had begun playing high school tennis, and he wasn't off to a good start. Although he was naturally athletic, Chris was a head case. He couldn't settle his nerves. While Julie's emotional makeup made for a more consistent tennis player who stayed cool under pressure and wore her opponent down, Chris was easily frustrated, often trying to kill the ball instead of returning it to his opponent. Due to his erratic play early in the season, I received instructions not to come to his first matches. But I ignored the warnings and went down one afternoon, hiding behind a car in the parking lot, wearing my bright red jacket and matching hat and gloves. It was a poor choice in colors. I was spotted, and Chris only got more distracted. By early April, Chris finally started to play more consistent tennis.

Midseason, I found out that one of the player's mothers had recently been diagnosed with fibromyalgia. She was "shattered" by the diagnosis, her words. I arranged to have lunch with her to share my over ten years of accumulated knowledge and provide some resources to help her live with the disease. Essentially, I compiled a layperson's survival guide to living with fibromyalgia. I prepared an entirely new diet and nutritional program for her, based on scientific findings. We focused on greatly restricting her carbohydrates and initially eliminating all simple sugar and yeast, both of which are shown to exacerbate the many symptoms of fibromyalgia, namely the diffuse muscle pain and fatigue.

My guide was also complete with web information and links to the various medications I had seen go through clinical trials and get FDA approval, such as Lyrica and Neurontin. Lyrica, in particular, showed great promise in treating the nerve pain associated with fibromyalgia, though I was yet to try it due to my usual fear of medicines. There were also links to holistic treatments to help manage fibromyalgia, including yoga, chiropractic treatment, massage, acupuncture, and other modalities. And finally, there was a very important reference to AAT, animal assisted therapy, with links supporting its efficacy, an avenue I had just begun to formally research myself despite being on the receiving end of pet therapy for years with my beloved rabbit. Caring for Bunny Boy—feeding him and changing his litter pan—kept me moving, which is critically important when you have fibromyalgia.

By this point, with my experience and keen interest in studying and understanding my diseases, I had become a wealth of information for new patients. I was honored that several rheumatologists felt confident enough to refer their fibromyalgia patients to me as a support system and guide. Fibromyalgia has no single definitive cause as of yet—just some solid theories—therefore, having an effective treatment plan can be complicated. Treatment usually encompasses mainstream medicine as well as a holistic approach, and often doctors do not have the time or capacity to provide comprehensive alternative medicine recommendations to their patients. That was where I came in.

Over the years, we had stacked up even more nicknames for Bunny Boy—Energizer Bunny, Happy Ears, Sunshine Boy, Pookie Doodles, or Butchie. But as of late, he was known as Iron Bunny, an endearment gifted upon him by Dr. Welch and enthusiastically supported by the Animal Medical Center. Bunny Boy had helped to teach the veterinarian community that indoor family rabbits can endure more medical procedures safely than they had previously believed. Bunny Boy had blazed a new trail for rabbits.

But having compromised immune systems set both him and me up for a myriad of annoying and sometimes life-threatening problems. By this point, we were routinely having Bunny Boy's molars and front teeth trimmed or his surface abscesses, which kept popping up, drained.

Between the two of us, I was not sure who spent more time at the doctor's. Around this time, I was dealing with my own health issues. While on Enbrel, I had used a corn pad on my right pinky toe. When the salicylic acid burned a hole through my skin to eliminate the corn, it also caused an infection. When on Enbrel, a simple infection can become problematic quickly, and this precipitated a ten-day round of antibiotics.

Additionally, despite brushing my pearly enamels three times a day, flossing rigorously, and rinsing my mouth with Listerine, my gums bled enough to send Ward running out of the bathroom. They had bled for years, another less common symptom of an autoimmune disease. *Chronic inflammation* was the term the doctors used, and anything could become inflamed, gums included. What I thought was a small inflamed pocket of skin over my eyetooth, which I noticed in the bathroom mirror one morning, turned out to be anything but. And Bunny Boy helped "discover" it.

I was lying on the sofa one afternoon, sulking over Julie's impending departure for college and Bunny Boy's aging. But Happy Ears wouldn't stand for it. He hopped onto my chest and swatted my face with his front paw, looking to play. When he drew his paw back, I noticed that it was bloody and that I had a nasty taste in my mouth. I looked in the mirror and the tiny bubble on my gum I had just seen early that morning was bleeding. It had grown to the size of a chickpea in a matter of hours. I snapped out of one funk and was thrown into another.

"We'll need to remove the growth," the gum specialist, Dr. Young, said, with an urgency that told me this was not simply a large pimple like I had initially assumed. "It might be a deep infection in the gum or the bone, or there's a chance it could be cancer."

I should have known better. I was aware that when you are on a powerful biologic like Enbrel or Humira, a small medical issue can turn into something life-threatening quickly. For the three days I waited to have the procedure, I couldn't eat or sleep. I told the children I had a small gum infection. There was no need to say more at the time. I also decided not to worry my mother or my siblings. Ward would be my strength. To get through those few days, I researched bone cancer on the Internet while the children were at school, and Bunny Boy stayed by my side almost constantly. I needed him near me, now more than ever.

The morning of the procedure, I got up, heavy with dread. I feared what the day would bring. The thought of cancer terrified me, but I knew Ward and I would face whatever it was together like we always did. The last thing I remembered was the bright light overhead as I sat in the chair and drifted off into semiconsciousness.

When I woke up from the anesthesia, Dr. Young was looking down at me. Ward was by his side.

"You didn't have cancer," he said, patting my shoulder. "But there was an abscess in the bone stemming from the root of your tooth."

I squeezed Ward's hand, wanting to cry. While I knew how dangerous a bone infection could be for me, at least I didn't have cancer!

He continued, "I implanted antibiotic beads into the bone that will release slowly over six months." My ears perked up. "It's a new procedure we're using in oral surgery."

His words were exact, his first sentence so familiar. For a split second I felt like I was back at the Animal Medical Center in New York. I had to speak up.

"Several years ago, our house rabbit, Bunny Boy, was one of the first mammals to have what sounds like similar antibiotic beads implanted in his jawbone at the Animal Medical Center in Manhattan," I exclaimed, suddenly wide awake. I was intrigued by what seemed to be another unbelievable coincidence, or just a plain old miracle. "Bunny Boy had a recurring chronic abscess and is immunocompromised. The veterinarian community believed that the beads, in addition to oral antibiotics and penicillin injections, could change the course of the very aggressive infection he had and that rabbits are prone to. Bunny Boy is alive and well, and a testament to that fact."

"Without the beads, the outcome might be very different in your case," said Dr. Young. The concern in his voice told me we were not completely out of the woods yet. "Once these infections are deep in the bone, they can go into the bloodstream, quickly causing septicemia." He didn't candy-coat his words. With a mother who was a nurse and my own keen interest in medicine, I knew exactly what septicemia was. It was often fatal.

"I would like to know more about your bunny's surgery at the Animal Medical Center when you are feeling a little better. I will make a call over to the AMC when I have a moment."

The revelation that I didn't have cancer, the miraculous coincidence of the antibiotic beads, and the stress that had been pent up over the last few days were too much for me. I released everything in tears of joy, while I quietly prayed. I thanked God for my life, my family, and my Bunny Boy, whose love and companionship had been such a godsend. I had yet to wrap my mind around the fact that Bunny Boy's groundbreaking treatment a few years ago had, amazingly, come full circle and helped save my life!

"Please stop in one day with Bunny Boy," said Dr. Young as he handed me a prescription for an antibiotic. "My partner, Dr. Pullman, has a particular affection for bunnies." Apparently, Dr. Pullman had a six-year-old rescue bunny named Flopsy, whom he adored.

"I'll see you at my post-op visit with Bunny Boy," I said, smiling.

• • •

Julie was due to leave very soon. In the lead-up to moving day, Bunny Boy and I were back to some of our old tricks, cruising the aisles of retail stores with Julie in tow for dorm room supplies and a new college wardrobe. Bunny Boy would sit in the top of the wagon at Marshalls or HomeGoods while we piled on our supplies.

While Julie and I ran up the credit cards, we reminisced about her younger years. The days of My Little Ponies and Care Bears, gymnastics lessons, and dance recitals. The days of ironing waxed paper onto beaded shapes for the neighbors' kids who played at our house almost daily. And finally, our time spent together in the Girl Scouts. I was halfway through a six-month protocol of gamma globulin infusions when Julie, who was in kindergarten, convinced me to run a Daisy/Brownie troop despite the fact that there had not been one in our town for the past eight years.

When the regional supervisor brought the troop flag and a pile of manuals over to our house a week later, she looked stunned when I answered the door with my intravenous pole trailing behind me.

"Are you sure you're up to this?" she asked hesitantly, staring at the vial of medicine.

I was lost in my memories.

Bunny Boy, I suspected, would feel Julie's loss profoundly, too. Julie hung out with him more than usual, telling him of her college plans and whispering, "I'm leaving home, little guy. I'll miss you, you know." Bunny Boy would nuzzle deep in her neck, tickling her with his whiskers. "Ooh, I'll miss that too. And take good care of Mom."

Chris, on the other hand, claimed he'd barely miss her. He liked the idea of having full access to the computer and food supply. But despite his strong statements, I sensed he was getting a little sentimental.

"Want to hit some tennis balls or get sushi, Jules?" he would ask. They would drive off in Julie's used bright red Honda Accord, which we had gotten for her sixteenth birthday, that suited her personality so well.

I, of course, would miss Julie with my whole heart. She was my first-born, and we had a special connection. Despite the usual challenges, we had made it through the teen years with very few issues or dramas. To soothe my upcoming loss, I would look through our baby albums, staring at Julie's pictures. Chris's accusations were not unfounded—there were many photos of Bunny Boy. Sadly, I realized how much he had aged. His cheeks were not as plump as they had once been and his fur had lost its thickness and brilliance.

Inspired by the photos, I came up with a wonderful idea. I chose two beautiful pictures of Bunny Boy, and together we went to CVS to get them printed on a coffee mug and a poster as gifts for Julie. While we were there, I also decided, on a whim, to order a deck of Bunny Boy–themed poker cards.

I broke out the keepsakes after dinner, the weekend before Julie left. Bunny Boy sat on my lap. I waited with bated breath as Julie reached into the colorful gift bag and unwrapped the coffee mug first.

"It's cute, Mom," she said in a monotone voice. Then she unrolled the poster. By that point, I would have been screaming, "Oh my god, I love it!" I had to stop trying to turn Julie into me!

"My roommate will think I'm crazy if I hang this!" she exclaimed.

I was heartbroken. "What about the coffee mug?" I managed to ask, through my hurt feelings.

"A beer mug might have been better," said Ward.

I tried to hide my disappointment, unsuccessfully. Julie handed me the poster and kissed my cheek.

"I'll use the mug for beer."

"Let's play a round of family poker with the cards, Mom," Chris said, putting his arm around me.

I scooped up Bunny Boy, looking for some affection, while Chris dealt the first hand. Playing poker with fifty-two pictures of Bunny Boy had to make me smile.

On moving day, Julie's bedroom lights were on by seven a.m. She and Bunny Boy were huddled under her lime-green comforter. Lime green had been her favorite color since she was seven years old, and if she wasn't dressed in lime-green clothing or lime-green high-top sneakers, she was cropping pictures of her friends into lime-green frames or threatening to wear a lime-green wedding dress when she got married.

As I stared at the teen magazines scattered on her bedroom floor and the celebrity posters on the walls, I wanted to throw my arms around her and tell her how much I loved her, but I was afraid I might cry. I had promised myself—and her—that I would keep it together. Life had passed right before my eyes, and my four-pound, thirteen-ounce baby girl had grown up to be a beautiful young lady. Like a mother bird, I knew it was time to let her fly. Julie was independent, cautious, sensible, poised, and a very intelligent woman ready to go out into the world. I was more worried about myself. My children were my life, and they gave me so much purpose. I prayed that once Chris left for college, too, that God would help me find purpose in the two difficult diseases I had been dealt.

Our fully loaded SUV pulled out of the driveway, sadly without Bunny Boy. It was eighty-five degrees outside, which was too hot for him. Besides, all hands were needed to haul and unpack Julie's belongings—her entire closet of clothes, two bureau drawers full of dorm wear and undies, and enough health and beauty aids for the entire dorm. We had to tie the trunk shut. I could hear Julie whisper affectionately out the open window of the car to Bunny Boy—"Goodbye, Stupid."

We drove the country route through the farmlands of central Jersey. You could see the mist coming up from the cornfields as the temperatures rose while the tractors toted their bales of hay. My thoughts wandered back to the days of hayrides or Halloween parties—when I dressed as a witch for Julie's kindergarten class and ladled blood (i.e., red Hi-C) out of my cauldron or sewed dolphin and Care Bear costumes. In the rearview mirror, Julie was glowing. She looked so ready for the next chapter of her life, with no apparent apprehension. Her natural confidence enveloped her. I knew we had done our job as parents.

Before I knew it, we had settled Julie in and it was time to leave.

Ward hugged her first. "Don't party too much and study hard, sweetheart."

Chris slapped her on the back. "Have fun, Sis."

Then it was my turn. The lump in my throat nearly choked me.

"I love you so much," I said, hugging her tightly. "I'm very proud of you, Juliebear. Stay safe and have fun."

And off Julie went, seemingly free as a bird, to join the other freshman students. Watching her retreating figure, I was reminded of her first day of nursery school when she strapped on her Care Bear backpack and walked away, not looking back.

On the ride home, I stared out the windshield for about a half hour and didn't speak. It was only when I saw the woman in the car we had been trailing since we left campus begin to cry that I started crying myself.

When we pulled into the driveway, I ran into the house, grabbed Bunny Boy off the sofa, and sobbed like a baby on Julie's bed, drenching her pillow and his fur. Bunny Boy stayed tucked under my armpit, intermittently poking his head up to lick my tears off the top of his head. One of the cutest things a rabbit does is when they try to groom their head—they lick their front paws while their ears drop to the side and duck their head down between their paws and scratch their head. It was the right amount of cuteness to plug my tears.

Ward walked by and peeked in. "You'll drown him, for Pete's sake, Nance."

Our bedroom door closed a minute later and the upstairs got quiet. Ward claimed he needed a nap, but I knew better.

Chapter 26

For the first few weeks that Julie was away, Bunny Boy sulked enough for the both of us. And he didn't hesitate to hop up the stairs to her bedroom, looking for someone he dearly missed. He would peer into her room from the hallway, and then sniff around her belongings and under her bed. He'd hop on the bed and sprawl out with his chin resting on her pillow. Somedays I would join him.

Autumn wasn't the same without Julie and her tennis matches. I yearned to host just one more pasta party with my silly tennis cake for her teammates. At home, there were no more sibling squabbles. The laundry was cut substantially, but I missed folding Julie's colorful, whimsical clothes, and Bunny Boy had to miss tossing her bras and underwear across her comforter, which he used to do if she left her clean laundry pile on the bed for too long.

Luckily, in no time at all, Julie was home for Thanksgiving. Bunny Boy seemed confused when she walked through the door. He sat on the kitchen chair for a minute, staring at her. But the moment he heard her voice, he lunged off and started binkying in a circle around her UGG boots until she picked him up and began singing to him.

We had our traditional Thanksgiving family gathering and cut down our Christmas trees on Saturday. The weekend was short and sweet. We drove Julie back to school on Sunday night, and Bunny Boy came along for the ride. He lay on Julie's lap the entire hour and a half, happy to have his number-two girl back—at least for a short while.

December felt like a whirlwind. Two more fibromyalgia patients were referred to me, this time from a rheumatologist who belonged to our tennis club and who had gotten my name from a friend. Helping these patients with a holistic program took up much of my time that was usually spent on holiday decorating and shopping. Ward was busy managing a new corporate client, and Chris was struggling to find his niche in high school. Was he a brainiac, a jock, or a party animal? He wanted to be all three. One night, to celebrate the end of his final exams, he spent a night out with his friends at a location undisclosed to us, returning home at one in the morning. We quickly established a curfew.

"It's too bad Bunny Boy can't bark," I said to Ward. "Then we could catch Chris coming home if we fall asleep."

A week before Christmas, the whole family regrouped again, watching *Die Hard* on our new flat screen television in the lagomorph lounge. It was wonderful to have everyone back together. Julie and Chris lay on the floor on a blanket and Bunny Boy hung out under our ten-foot weeping white pine, which glistened with lights, reflecting off the large picture window.

I wasn't expecting it to happen. During a commercial break, I went down to the kitchen to make some popcorn, and when I returned, Bunny Boy lunged onto my lap, nearly knocking over the bowl of popcorn. He was clenching one of my favorite Christmas ornaments in his crooked teeth, a hand-painted nativity scene. I cupped his face to pry it loose and instantly felt sick.

"Bunny Boy has two abscesses on his jaw," I shrieked. "One on each side." I could feel they were attached to the bone. They were not surface abscesses. Heartbroken, I phoned the Animal Medical Center's emergency line and scheduled an appointment for the following morning.

Bunny Boy and I went into the city alone that Saturday. I wanted it that way, though I wasn't sure why. The news was bad. Both abscesses were already in the bone and there was significant scar tissue on one side. Bunny Boy would need extensive surgery, which meant more anesthesia. My biggest concern was his age—Bunny Boy was seven years old. But after a thorough examination and consultation at the AMC, Dr. Quesenberry, the new exotics veterinarian, assured me that Bunny Boy's vital signs and overall health seemed good.

"I will draw some blood to make sure Bunny Boy's organs are functioning properly," she said, looking at his chart. "I read the notes here and spoke to a few of our veterinarians. It seems Bunny Boy's well-known around here. I couldn't wait to meet him."

It was true. I had just received another call from the hospital requesting permission to use his records for a teaching seminar.

I left the hospital, heavy with dread. I drove across town, going up Fifth Avenue and heading to the Henry Hudson Parkway along the Hudson River for a change of scenery. I was unable to fully appreciate the magic of the city at Christmas time—the horse-drawn carriages filled with tourists, the thousands of white lights that lined the streets, and the spectacular holiday window displays on both sides of Fifth Avenue. Having to make the decision about whether or not to let Bunny Boy have the surgery weighed heavy on my mind.

When I spotted a large clock on one of the Trump towers that said one o'clock, I remembered that Dr. Welch was usually in her office until two on Saturdays. If I picked up my speed, I could make it there before she left for the day. Dr. Welch knew Bunny Boy better than anyone else from a medical standpoint. She would know whether or not he was strong enough for surgery.

We pulled into the mini mall in front of Dr. Welch's office just minutes before two. The parking lot was jammed with cars, many of them stationed outside of parking spaces. I was puzzled. There were no other retail stores around to attract holiday shoppers. I joined the other lawbreaking citizens, parking alongside a large dumpster. There was a sign on the door of the animal hospital.

"Pet photos with Santa, December 16."

Bunny Boy and I squeezed our way into the crowded lobby. Every owner of a dog or cat from the county must have showed up. A brown Yorkie was slumped over from the weight of his reindeer antlers, two chocolate Labradors were dressed as Mr. and Mrs. Claus, and a white poodle had a red plaid bow around her neck and bells around her ankles. There was even a giant black Bernese mountain dog dressed as a snowman. Christmas music was pumping through the speakers and the hospital staff was dressed in holiday attire, as were many of the pet owners. I immediately felt happier.

"There's Bunny Boy!" shrieked Kelly, pushing through the crowd to get to us. Kat and Donna, two other technicians, who were sipping hot cider and policing the long line of pets, also spotted us. "It's Bunny Boy," they yelled over the noise of the crowd. He was a celebrity.

Dr. Welch walked over, wearing a red turtleneck and a Santa hat. She threw her arms around me. Her warmth and brilliant smile were just what I needed.

"We're so glad to see Bunny Boy this year," she said, playing with his nose.

Careful not to put a damper on the festive mood, I took Dr. Welch aside and told her about Bunny Boy's situation.

"Bunny Boy's a very strong rabbit, Mrs. Laracy," she said, flashing me her most reassuring smile. "His spirit is remarkable." As always, I knew she was right.

"Let's wait to see what the bloodwork shows. In the meantime, let's see if we can get you bumped to the front of the line, Bunny Boy. You've both had a rough morning." She grabbed my hand and gently guided me through the crowd.

Sheepishly, I walked over toward Santa and handed him Bunny Boy.

"Ho ho ho," Santa rumbled. "I believe you're my first rabbit this season."

"Here, put this on Bunny Boy!" exclaimed Kelly, handing Santa a small Santa hat for Bunny Boy.

As the flash went off, I made my decision. Bunny Boy would have the surgery after the holidays, god willing, if all of his blood work came up fine.

Even without a costume, Bunny Boy was a great attraction for the pet owners patiently waiting in line. I stood cradling him, complimenting owners on their pets and costumes while answering questions about lagomorphs and dispelling some myths about the species.

"You should write a book about Bunny Boy, Mrs. Laracy," said Dr. Welch. "Bunny Boy's the unluckiest, but luckiest, rabbit in the world. He may have been born with seemingly insurmountable health issues, but he found his way into your family. Your love and strength has kept him fighting. We've all been witness to your remarkable journey and the bond you and Bunny Boy have formed."

"We'll have a book signing right here!" Kelly suggested.

I looked at the bookshelves filled with pet books for sale and thought, *Yes! I will write a book!* It would be part of the next chapter of my life. It would be about Bunny Boy and me, and it would inspire people suffering with any sickness or disease. It would be a story of resilience and bravery.

Despite my deep worries, I walked out into the cold, feeling a renewed sense of hope and merriment.

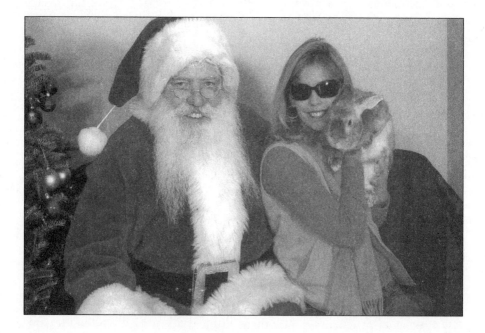

Chapter 27

The results of Bunny Boy's blood work came back after the New Year. Our geriatric bunny had the liver and kidney function of a much younger rabbit. The surgery was on. But there was a change in plans. Bunny Boy had several infected teeth near the abscesses that needed to be pulled out, and his molars needed to be trimmed again. The dental work, together with the surgery, would require too much anesthesia over a long period of time. Dr. Quesenberry wanted to do the procedures separately, feeling it was a safer option for Bunny Boy. But I worried that administering anesthesia twice in two weeks would be too much for Bunny Boy. I would turn out to be right.

The snow was coming down heavy by the time I arrived in the city for Bunny Boy's dental work. Pedestrians pulled their hoods tight as the wind howled and the snow swirled up First Avenue along the water.

"It's D-Day, Bunny Boy," I said, pushing the elevator button. "By this time tomorrow, you'll have a whole new mouth." The elevator stopped on the third floor and a group of interns stepped in, carrying their trays of coffee.

"Is that Bunny Boy?" one of them suddenly asked, catching me by surprise. Bunny Boy was resting on my chest with his head on my shoulder.

"Yes, he is! I'm Mrs. Laracy." I reached my hand out to shake one of their hands.

"We just sat through a lecture three weeks ago regarding innovative breakthroughs in animal medicine. Bunny Boy's records were discussed with regard to bunny dental care." Of course, I already knew that; I had received the call.

I felt a sense of pride and accomplishment for Bunny Boy. "Bunny Boy helped save my life," I said, kissing Bunny Boy's cheek. "I was the grateful recipient of his cutting-edge treatment—the antibiotic beads."

Their interest was immediately piqued. We got off the elevator together and I quickly told them my story before we checked in.

Coming out of the anesthesia seemed more difficult for Bunny Boy this time. The surgeon used Ketamine for the surgery, and Dr. Quesenberry warned me that Bunny Boy's body would be stiff for a while. While it was unnerving to see no warmth or movement in his body, his shallow breathing upset me the most. Wrapped in a blanket, Bunny Boy slept in my arms the entire first night home, barely moving.

"Mommy's here, Bunny Boy," I kept whispering into his drooped ears. "You're going to feel better tomorrow." I almost called Dr. Welch for assurance that Bunny Boy's reaction to the anesthesia was normal. My gut told me it was not.

By mid-morning the following day, Bunny Boy's muscles had softened and he was more alert, but he showed very little interest in anything but resting. And unlike the last few times in the past, he wasn't the least bit excited to eat his critical care food. My instincts told me he needed more time to recover between surgeries—and if only I had listened to myself.

Bunny Boy went into cardiac arrest on the operating table the following week. For the first time, I wasn't there waiting in the lobby. Chris had taken a bad fall in the gym at school, and I had been called back to New Jersey during his surgery.

Dr. Quesenberry's voice was serious but calm over the phone.

"We were able to resuscitate Bunny Boy, but we had to close the wounds up before we could clean out the abscesses. We can rarely resuscitate a rabbit, Mrs. Laracy. His condition is grave."

I nearly dropped my cell phone. I could barely respond. I felt like I had been hit over the head with a brick. Bunny Boy had survived so much—like a cat. I'd always assumed he had nine lives.

"I'll do everything that's possible for Bunny Boy," said Dr. Quesenberry. "When can I expect you, Mrs. Laracy?" I was filled with an overwhelming sense of helplessness, being so far away. I was also torn about leaving Chris, who, though very shaken up, seemed okay.

"We'll keep an eye on, Chris," mouthed the school nurse. "You do what you need to do."

I called Ward, who agreed without hesitation to join me at the recovery room to be with Bunny Boy. My sister, Carol, would take care of Chris. We made it into the city from New Jersey in less than forty minutes. On the tense ride over, the muscle spasms in my back and neck, which were already painful, intensified. It felt like a vicelike grip was strangling my spinal column. I wished I'd had the time to pick up my battery-operated TENS unit that I had started using the past year under the recommendation of my chiropractor, whom I saw almost weekly. When the back pain was unbearable, I would hook the cell phone–size unit to the waist of my pants, stick the electrodes on, and wear it all day. It dulled the pain significantly, helping me go on with my life. When we reached the AMC, instead of waiting for the elevator, we ran up the stairs. I charged the desk.

"Bunny Boy Laracy," I exclaimed, half out of breath. "Dr. Quesenberry is expecting me." An intern led us to the recovery room where she was waiting for us. "His heart has been stressed," she said. "But he is resting comfortably."

Fear and sadness enveloped me. Had I expected too much of Bunny Boy? Had his body been through enough? He was stiff and motionless, and his usually big and beautiful eyes were barely open. His nose looked dry, and his breathing was shallow. My gut churned. My lips were bitten and scratched up from the stress. As I stared at my boy, almost afraid to touch him, I worried I had made the wrong decision to go ahead with the surgery. But somehow I knew my boy was still there.

I leaned down and kissed Bunny Boy's shaven face. Bunny Boy was fighting to stay alive. I was sure—for both of us. My hands started trembling as I softly petted the top of his head. "I love you, little man. Don't give up, please," I begged. I could feel my tears building up. Remarkably, Bunny Boy's still whiskers suddenly started to flutter gently and his pale nose began to twitter. My bunny vital signs.

"Bunny Boy definitely knows you're his mommy," said Dr. Quesenberry, clenching my hand.

"We call him Iron Bunny," added Ward, kissing Bunny Boy's head tenderly.

"Let's try to get Bunny Boy stable. We'll talk again in a few hours," Dr. Quesenberry finally suggested, wrapping her arm around my shoulder. It was time for us to leave.

I melted into Ward's arms. The fear inside of me was bigger than I could handle. I wasn't ready to lose Bunny Boy.

By this point, my back and neck pain were intolerable. Burning nerve pain was shooting down my legs. Sitting in a hard, plastic chair in the hospital's waiting room would be difficult, so we walked to the hotel next door and sat on a tufted sofa in a quiet, dimly lit corner of the room. I needed to keep up my own strength in order to take care of Bunny Boy. Ward had a much-needed beer while I took four Advil tablets, for inflammation, and one .25 mg Xanax for the nerve pain—a combination of meds that, over the years, I had found relieved the pain better than anything else. I laid on Ward's lap and whimpered like a wounded puppy dog. A waitress at the hotel tried to make small talk but quickly realized we wanted to be alone. My cellphone buzzed at ten thirty. We were being called back.

Bunny Boy's breathing was still shallow and irregular. He was listless.

"It's going to take time," Dr. Quesenberry reassured us. "Bunny Boy's been through a lot. It's a miracle he's still with us."

There were a few more preparations they had to make, so Ward and I went out to the lobby to wait again. I prayed fervently to God. *Don't take Bunny Boy, not yet.* I wasn't ready. I thought about what life would be like without him. All the things I would miss. His warm, furry body. His twittering nose. His loving, steadfast companionship. His zest for life. I smiled, thinking about the time he challenged the squirrel or the time he rolled upside down in the PVC pipe. I marveled at the day he nudged the phone over to me while I lay semi-paralyzed on my bed. I cringed, remembering the time he broke his jaw and the time he hopped on my foot on the gas pedal, nearly killing us both.

Two hours passed. Then three. We sat in silence. I was distracted, lost in thought, when I heard, "I think this little guy is ready to go home."

Dr. Quesenberry was standing beside us, holding a bundle in her arms. She looked relaxed. Bunny Boy's beautiful head was peering out of a blue plaid blanket. I thought I would burst with joy.

"Bunny Boy's vital signs are good. I think he belongs at home with you now."

"Are you sure?"

I had assumed Bunny Boy would be staying overnight in the hospital. I was terrified to bring him home, so far away from medical care should something happen.

"Rabbits do not do well alone, caged in a strange place overnight. We avoid that at all costs. Often, we do keep them here, but right now I believe Bunny Boy and his heart would be less stressed at home with you."

A rush of emotion came over me. "I'm sorry I wasn't here, buddy," I said, apologizing. "Chris needed me. I love you so much, Bunny Boy." Tears spilled down my cheeks. Dr. Quesenberry watched as Bunny Boy lifted his head ever so slightly and gazed up at me.

"Bunny Boy is so strong, Mrs. Laracy, because he is so loved. That's apparent. His will to survive surpasses anything I've ever seen in a bunny."

I tried to acknowledge her kind words with a simple, "Thank you."

We walked down the hallway toward the checkout counter. It was one in the morning. Ward greeted the cashier in a cheerful tone, despite the ungodly hour and everything we had been through. The bill was two pages long, totaling nineteen hundred dollars. Ward checked over each item carefully, unlike myself who, at that point, would have rolled it up and stuffed it in my purse without a second glance. I was exhausted, and I just wanted to get home with Bunny Boy.

"So, let me get this straight," he said to the cashier, "Bunny Boy died temporarily, and now you are charging me $250 to do CPR on a rabbit? For that amount of money, I want a demonstration."

The woman started scrolling down anxiously on her computer screen, trying to find that specific charge. "If you just give me a second, I can find—"

"I was just joking," Ward said, cracking a smile. "We are so grateful to the veterinarians that Bunny Boy is still alive. We knew the risks."

We should have insisted on the demonstration. A year and a half later, we would need it.

• • •

Once again, Iron Bunny had survived a near-death experience. Nothing kept him down for long. He recovered from this anesthesia quickly and ate his critical care food happily, propped in my left arm while I pushed the syringe with my right, just like I was feeding a baby. Bunny Boy's head would bob forward, much like Julie's would when I fed her, and his thumper feet would pump back and forth with excitement, nearly hitting me on the nose. Between the apple banana goop and the new cotton candy–flavored antibiotic from the compounding pharmacy, Bunny Boy binkied around the house with a lightheartedness I wished I could feel, too.

But how could I? Without the success of the surgery, our time with Bunny Boy would be short. While my muscle pain had subsided after Bunny Boy's ordeal, the emotional pain I felt was growing. I refused to speak about it to Ward or the children. We resumed our routine, giving Bunny Boy his penicillin shots and the oral antibiotic and doing hot compresses. This time I used one of my own heat wraps, which fit around his entire jaw, making him look like one of those people wearing a neck brace after a car accident—except for the tall ears!

I met with Dr. Welch once Bunny Boy was able to eat his pellets again. Bunny Boy was back—which I was able to confirm when he sprayed me! I told her the harrowing details of both surgeries.

"You said they were unable to remove the abscesses before Bunny Boy went into cardiac arrest, correct?" she said, looking at me quizzically.

"Yes, that's right."

She relit her scope and examined the inside of Bunny Boy's mouth. Then she palpated both sides of Bunny Boy's jaw blindly, numerous times.

"Feel right here, Mrs. Laracy"

Dr. Welch took my hands and clasped them around Bunny Boy's jaw. There was just one small band of what felt like tight elastic on the side where he had had his previous surgery. That was all.

"Both of the abscesses are gone," she remarked, as if she couldn't believe it herself. "There's just scar tissue on the one side."

"Are you sure?" I gasped.

"I'm sure." She tilted her head, looking up at me with a crooked smile as if to say, "Are *you* surprised?" I grabbed Bunny Boy off the table and started dancing around the room.

"It's a miracle, Dr. Welch."

How could the antibiotics alone have gotten rid of the abscesses?

"Bunny Boy's one big miracle," said Dr. Welch. "I won't question anything when it comes to him."

Bunny Boy had pulled off a hat trick. He had survived cardiac arrest and two abscesses. But I couldn't help but wonder if his bunny luck was beginning to run out.

Chapter 28

Julie was thriving at college. She had made the dean's list her first semester and joined Phi Sigma Sigma sorority. Greek life, which I knew very little about, involved numerous community projects like working at the food bank nearby and mentoring local high school students, much to my pleasant surprise. I was proud of her. She was following in her grandmother's footsteps.

While I had looked forward to having Julie around for the summer, much to our disappointment, she had found herself a job working as a counselor at a sleepaway camp in Pennsylvania. Most of my summer was spent instead at our club pool on a chaise lounge under an umbrella, drafting an outline for my book about Bunny Boy and me, which was beginning to take shape. I had begun expanding my networking and contacts among the national pain community in the past year, including the National Fibromyalgia and Chronic Pain Association (NFMCPA) and the World Institute of Pain (WIP). The chronic pain and disease community, along with the pet community, was my target audience for the book.

One day in early August, a jellybean-sized lump next to Bunny Boy's nose sent us back to visit our friends at the Franklin Lakes Animal Hospital.

"It's not much more than a big pimple," Dr. Welch remarked. She sounded as relieved as I felt. Since we were there, Dr. Welch searched Bunny Boy's body for possible new abscesses, finding nothing except for some tiny brown specks buried deep in his fur—flea droppings. Half-jokingly, she assumed a look as though she were afraid to tell me the bad news.

"The pampered prince has fleas, Mrs. Laracy," she blurted out, covering her mouth to suppress her laughter.

"Fleas? That's impossible." I said as she separated his fur into sections and showed me the droppings.

"Has Bunny Boy been outside in the grass lately?" she asked.

"Not that I'm aware of," I replied. I raised my eyebrows, and my mind wandered to Chris. Though I had only caught him once, I suspected he might have snuck Bunny Boy outside periodically without my knowledge.

"Have there been any other pets in your home recently?"

"Not that I'm aware of," I repeated.

I sounded like a politician being interrogated by the Senate committee. "What on earth do I do now?"

"You'll need to bomb every room in the house where Bunny Boy spends time with special chemicals. You can buy them at any pet store."

Bunny Boy was sitting upright on the table with his ears in their "happy" position, completely oblivious to his critter infestation. "Should I buy one of those flea collars?"

"Flea collars are too dangerous for rabbits. You'll have to comb his fur with rubbing alcohol to get rid of the fleas, though I don't see any at the moment. Good luck catching the fleas, Mrs. Laracy," she said in jest, handing me a small green comb with metal teeth. "This might be your biggest challenge yet. The comb's a little present for Bunny Boy."

I phoned Ward from the car.

"Did you say Bunny Boy has fleas?"

"I did. It's ridiculous, isn't it?"

"I can't wait to tell Gregory about this one. So what's the plan?"

"I have to bomb the house with chemicals."

"With us in it?"

"I have no idea yet."

"Just tell me when it's safe to come home," he joked.

At Scuffy's, I purchased rubbing alcohol and enough chemicals to clear out any mosquitoes that our Mosquito Magnet missed. I felt a surge of silliness when I told Loretta about the fleas.

Once home, I set up shop in the green bathroom upstairs. Bunny Boy scratched his ears with his hind paws, and I wondered if he was feeling itchy from the fleas. I separated the first small section of Bunny Boy's fur, dipped the comb in the bowl of rubbing alcohol, and ran it through slowly. All I found were flea droppings. Stationary brown specks, not moving ones. Bunny Boy sat on my lap contently, probably thinking it was just another type of spa treatment.

I dipped and combed, dipped and combed. But there were still no fleas. By the seventh sequence, Bunny Boy and I were both getting impatient. He kept trying to knock away the comb and lick his fur at the same time, which made my job harder. I cursed under my breath.

"How's it going in there?" asked Chris, peeking into the bathroom. "You sound a little frustrated, Mom!"

"I haven't spotted a single flea," I replied, exasperated. "Just their droppings."

"If anyone can catch and eradicate them, it's you, Nancinator. Just keep your cool."

I was particularly fond of the nickname. It was about as endearing as I could expect from my teenage male offspring.

"Want to give me a hand?" I asked with a pitiful look on my face.

"Hey Jules, we could use some help in the green bathroom," he yelled downstairs. Although she had been away for most of the summer, Julie had returned and would be staying with us for six weeks before her next semester started. The three of us launched a full-scale invasion of Bunny Boy's fur. He fought us like a boxer in training, swinging at us with his front paws. Eventually, we turned up one lone flea. I whisked the comb under the tiny critter and flushed him down the toilet.

I bombed the house the next morning and we spent the day at my mother's. Her poor cats were locked behind a gate upstairs while the prince had full run of her house.

Chris never owned up to bringing Bunny Boy outside. But I knew better.

I was the next to turn fifty soon. I felt optimistic and happy. Life was good. My health was stable for the time being, my children were flourishing, and Bunny Boy had filled the void I had felt over not having a third child. He completed our family.

Six weeks before my milestone birthday, Ward and I were hanging out in the sunroom with our best friends. We would be having dinner at a Caribbean restaurant later that evening and were pregaming on margaritas with cute umbrellas in them and fresh fruit stuffed in a hollowed-out pineapple. Bunny Boy hopped onto my lap, a pink umbrella in his teeth, just as music came blaring through the speakers behind the bar—"Margaritaville" by Jimmy Buffett.

"Surprise!" everyone announced. "We're going to St. Thomas next week!"

I was completely surprised—and ecstatic.

Ward had arranged everything. My brother, Jack, would keep an eye on Chris, and Kelly would visit with penicillin injections for Bunny Boy every other day. He would be on the shots for the remainder of his life.

We spent our time in St. Thomas decompressing, as I liked to call it—soaking up the sun at the pool and the beach and simply relaxing. I called home every day to check on Bunny Boy and Chris. On the fourth day, we sailed for eight hours through the crystal-clear blue waters of the Caribbean while steel drum music played softly in the background. Our first stop was St. John, where we snorkeled in a scenic cove along Honeymoon Beach. Next, we sailed to Virgin Gorda and disembarked for an hour to shop at the small stores along the pier. When we reboarded, the captain took us to Jost Van Dyke, where we paddled our way to shore on Styrofoam floats and enjoyed drinks at the famous Soggy Dollar Bar. Except for a few drops of rain on the first day and a delayed flight during the tail end of our trip, our island getaway was magical.

Around this time, Bunny Boy had also turned eight years old. It was an important birthday for our lagomorph. He had lived to his full life expectancy—seven to eight years. We made a bigger fuss than normal. I baked a bunny cake and filled a dozen mini bunny molds, which were sitting in a tray, with timothy hay pellets. Bunny Boy flipped the tray over almost immediately. It was the thought that counted.

A few days after his birthday, I was invited to a "Girls' Night Out" at a local Italian Restaurant, which ended up being another surprise party for me. There wasn't a single detail my devoted girlfriends had overlooked.

There were lavender and pink flowers in black glass cubes on the tables, a luscious buffet of Italian specialties, a hysterical roasting of the guest of honor, and a massive collage with embarrassing photos of my entire life on display. Out of the fifty-plus photos of my family and me, Bunny Boy was in at least a dozen. It was special night I would never forget.

I barely had time to send out thank you cards before our Christmas party approached. I could not help but continue to be in the most festive of moods, considering all the celebrating that had taken place. Bunny Boy was the pampered prince, and I truly felt like his pampered princess. During the party, Bunny Boy wore his Santa hat and I donned a tiara with gold stones that read "Fifty." I wasn't sure I was deserving of so much love and attention.

As the icing on the cake, my baby brother, Tom, and his family arrived from Colorado in time to celebrate Christmas. It was the only gift I had asked for.

While I caught up with my sister-in-law, Audrey, and the boys, Tom wasted no time rekindling his relationship with Bunny Boy, lying on the rug face to face with our bunny and talking to him softly.

"I gotta tell you, you're really something else, Bunny Boy," he'd say. "I would have never thought a rabbit could bring such love to a house like you do. Your mother's crazy about you." With his loving, affectionate nature and stoicism in the face of adversity, Bunny Boy had won the hearts and respect of my entire family. For the first time in fifteen years, the entire Buchalski family rocked under one roof on Christmas Eve in a boisterous, emotion-filled celebration of twenty-four close relatives. My mother was beaming. There was nothing that meant more to her than her family—just as it did to me.

Fifty, for me, was a wonderful place to be.

Chapter 29

In a few months, I had gone from being on top of the world to teetering on the edge of exhaustion. My mother was having a myriad of medical problems that required my attention, which I gladly gave her. Chris and I were arguing regularly over how much time was appropriate to spend on homework versus electronic games. He seemed to think that, once he hit six feet tall, I couldn't tell him what to do. Often, he would sit on the couch with Bunny Boy and play Halo or World of Warcraft until he developed calluses on his fingers. On top of being the auction committee chairman for a large charity event for pediatric cancer, which required me calling in favors from anyone unlucky enough to have crossed my path—often from my bed or the sofa because the pain and malaise had become debilitating again—I was also working with a few new fibromyalgia patients who had been referred to me. Soon, I was beginning to feel that the load on my back was too heavy. When Bunny Boy's facial abscess came back, this time much larger than before, despite his prophylactic penicillin injections, I felt ready to burst.

Then the house phone rang.

It was a reporter from the *Suburban News*, a widely circulated newspaper in our area. She wanted to do a feature story on Bunny Boy for Easter. I was flattered and euphoric. It was our first chance to share our story publicly and hopefully inspire those suffering with chronic illness.

"You're going to be a celebrity, pal," I told him.

The reporter, Jenny, showed up promptly with her briefcase and notepad. She greeted us warmly but didn't seem the least bit surprised to see a house bunny. Of course, she had been given the whole backstory. We spoke about rabbits as a species—their habits, food preferences, and traits. We talked specifically about Bunny Boy, his health issues, and his place in our family. Then, we talked about my own health and how it was so intertwined with Bunny Boy's. Jenny asked pointed questions and jotted down notes while Bunny Boy sat on my lap, keenly interested in her. He kept leaning forward to sniff her blazer. I didn't find out until after the interview that she had yogurt drops for Bunny Boy in her pocket. Finally, we moved to the sunroom for a couple of photographs.

"Bunny Boy inspires me," I said at the close of the interview, giving him a look of adoration. "I hope other people will be inspired by and find strength from our story. Bunny Boy has shown me that unconditional love heals. It prolongs life. We have both shown each other that."

The following week, I stopped by my church for a visit. The assistant at the rectory was holding the *Suburban News* as I walked in. She looked at me as if she had seen a ghost.

"You're on the cover of the newspaper, Mrs. Laracy!" she exclaimed.

There we were, on the cover, Bunny Boy and I gazing into each other's eyes like two lovers. The headline read: "He Makes Her Heart Go Hippity Hop." The picture and article took up most of the front page, and an interview with Dina, one of the stars of the new upcoming television series "The Real Housewives of New Jersey," was squeezed to the far-left corner of the front page. I was told that Bravo, the TV series' production company, wasn't happy. I should have realized what she meant when she said "feature story."

The story was beautifully written and informative. Jenny gave a brief overview of the lagomorph species, then focused on Bunny Boy's health issues and his role in pioneering a medical treatment that helped save my life. Finally, she described my intimate moments with Bunny Boy. "The bond between Mrs. Laracy and Bunny Boy grew in sickness and in health," she eloquently wrote.

Bunny Boy's story could now touch many people's lives. And this was just the beginning.

•   •   •

One day, when I stopped over unannounced to visit my mother, I found her lying in bed, burning up with a fever. She seemed confused as to who I was. Carol had left her alone at home only the day before to visit friends in South Carolina. The ambulance showed up within four minutes of my frantic phone call.

When she was eighty, my mother's health had started to deteriorate rapidly. She had high blood pressure, and her potassium, sodium, and calcium levels were fluctuating erratically, often becoming too low, which the geriatrics doctor diagnosed as hyponatremia, a condition commonly seen in the elderly. She was also plagued with urinary tract infections, which were common among the older community. I quickly learned that UTIs could cause delirium in elderly people.

Upon arrival at the hospital, it was confirmed that she was suffering from delirium caused by a UTI that had entered her bloodstream. My brothers Mike and Jack met me in the emergency room. She had septicemia, a bloodstream infection, which was often fatal. Carol rushed home from South Carolina and Tom flew in from Colorado. All five siblings gathered around my mother's bedside for almost a week as she fought the battle of her life.

One night, Tom and I returned home from the hospital around eleven thirty, tired and emotionally drained. Amid the stress and distractions of the past few hours, I suddenly remembered it was the alternate day—Bunny Boy would need his penicillin shot. It was Ward's chance to impress my baby brother, who was a nurse, with his injecting skills. We gathered around as Ward placed Bunny Boy on the kitchen counter and inserted the needle, as he always had.

As the needle sunk into the skin, Bunny Boy suddenly collapsed. He slumped down onto his belly, his front paws splaying forward and his back legs trailing out behind him. He looked as if he were about to belly crawl off the counter. I leapt forward and picked him up. His body was heavy, and he hung limp against me, almost dangling.

"Something's wrong," I screeched, clutching him against my chest. "Something's horribly wrong!"

"Lay him on the counter," Tom said firmly but calmly. Trembling, I laid Bunny Boy down on his side. I looked on in horror as Bunny Boy's eyes closed—and then he stopped breathing.

"My god, what's happening, Tom?" I screamed loudly.

"The closest vet is over half of an hour away!" Ward told Tom, hovering over Bunny Boy.

"There's no time for a vet," said Tom with urgency. I knew instantly that this was a matter of life or death. I laid my head on Bunny Boy's chest and started crying. Had he had a heart attack?

"I'm so sorry, Bunny Boy. I'm so sorry, buddy," I blubbered through my tears. "I'm right here."

"Do you have any oxygen in the house?" Tom asked quickly.

"Why would we have oxygen in the house?" I snapped back, immediately regretting my tone, which I had no control over. "Please, God, don't take Bunny Boy now," I prayed, hanging onto his limp body. "Don't take my boy. I can't handle anymore right now."

"Squire, get her off of him," Tom demanded, using Ward's nickname. Chris, who had come down from his bedroom after hearing the commotion, stood rigid as he watched the awful scene unfold, not uttering a single word, in total disbelief. For years, Chris had seen his father give Bunny Boy his injections without incident.

I stepped back and let Tom take charge. He grabbed Ward's elbow. "Stand here. I'll need you to do the chest compressions."

Tom placed his mouth over Bunny Boy's snout and started blowing air into his lungs while using his hands to push lightly on Bunny Boy's chest.

"Like this," Tom told Ward.

Together, they began administering CPR.

"C'mon, little buddy. C'mon, little buddy." Tom blew another rescue breath into Bunny Boy. "Ready, Squire—again."

Tom blew another breath; Ward did another compression. Bunny Boy showed no sign of life.

"C'mon, little buddy! C'mon, little buddy!" Tom repeated, shaking Bunny Boy, trying to stimulate his heart. Tom blew his fourth rescue breath.

"Hang in there, Bunny Boy!" His voice was getting louder and more stressed. "Again, Squire!" Desperately, Tom breathed more air into Bunny Boy's lungs.

"Let's go, Bunny Boy, gosh darnit. You're not leaving us yet," Tom yelled, as I cried out again, "God, please don't take Bunny Boy. I'm not ready."

Suddenly, Tom signaled for Ward to step back. In a horrible split second, I thought Tom had given up. Instead, he laid his head on Bunny Boy's chest. Then I knew by the look of sheer relief and emotion on his face that he had heard the first beats of Bunny Boy's heart. I gasped—Bunny Boy had opened his eyes.

"I can feel his breath against my cheek. It's shallow, but it's there." Tom sighed, his head still flush against Bunny Boy's chest. "Step back," he whispered. "Give Bunny Boy some space." Slowly, Bunny Boy's chest rose and receded, rose and receded. Tom stood up.

"Pick Bunny Boy up and put him against your chest, sis. We need to keep him warm. Go get a blanket, Chris."

As Chris scrambled off, I leaned my head on Tom's shoulder. Beads of perspiration dripped down his temple. "Thank god you were here, Tom," I whimpered.

Ward didn't look much better. "I've given Bunny Boy that shot on and off for years and—" he started, shaken.

Tom wrapped his arm around Ward's shoulder. "You gave him a text-book shot, Squire. But the needle must have hit a vein. The penicillin went straight to Bunny Boy's heart. It can happen to anyone. I've seen it happen at my hospital."

Time stood still for us over the next hour. We sat quietly on the family room sofas, trying to process what had just happened.

"Was he dead, Uncle Tom?" Chris asked, hesitantly.

"Bunny Boy's heart had stopped beating, Chris."

"What should I expect now?" I asked my brother.

Bunny Boy was lying on my chest, wrapped in the blanket. His ears were ice cold and lying flat on top of his head. He seemed spooked. His head flicked from side to side, but his body remained perfectly still. I was concerned that he had sustained brain damage from the lack of oxygen for what had seemed to me like an immeasurable amount of time, though it had probably been only about two minutes. Tom had worked fast, with Ward playing a vital role. I, on the other hand, had been useless. And I wasn't proud of that. It wasn't like me to panic under stress. When a crisis arose or an accident happened involving the children—and there had been many over the years—I had always kept my cool and worked quickly to get the necessary help or solve the problem myself.

"These next few hours are critical," Tom said in a somber tone.

None of us left the room. We sat quietly with Bunny Boy, listening to soft, relaxing music on the television for about an hour. Finally, Tom told us to put Bunny Boy down on the floor. I watched in anguish as Bunny Boy struggled to stand up.

"It's okay, pal." I said, bracing his hips. "Everything is going to be fine."

When he tried to hop, his hind legs dragged behind him. I thought I might get sick. "Is he paralyzed?" I asked.

"More than likely it's temporary, Nance."

I lay down on the carpet and started coaxing him. "Come on, Bunny Boy," I said, reaching my arms out. "You can do it."

As if he didn't want to let me down, Bunny Boy crawled painfully toward me and climbed onto my torso, his legs trailing behind him, jerking involuntarily.

Tom finally let it all out. "In all my years of medicine, I've rarely felt as stressed as when I performed rescue breathing on Bunny Boy. I'd like to go out to the garage to have a cigarette now, if nobody minds. Actually, maybe two or three."

"I'll join," said Ward, though he was not a smoker.

When they returned, Ward tried to break the somber mood. "I should have insisted on the CPR demonstration at the Animal Medical Center, Nance." He turned to Tom to explain. "Bunny Boy's had CPR before. We almost lost him on the operating table during his last surgery."

By around two in the morning, Bunny Boy had regained full use of his hind legs, and his involuntary jerking motions subsided.

"Go try to get some rest, Tom," I said, giving him a big hug. "You have an early flight out tomorrow. We can handle things from here."

My baby brother walked up the stairs toward the guest bedroom, then stopped in the hallway and looked back at me. "By the way, sis, did I earn a chapter in your book?"

"My god, of course you did!"

Chapter 30

After six long, grueling weeks in the hospital, our matriarch, who was now bedridden and had to be fed through a gastric tube, was finally transferred to a rehabilitation facility. Despite surviving septicemia, she had suffered mini strokes and developed several dangerous infections, which had damaged her aging brain and prolonged her hospital stay. But Mom was a fighter.

The rehabilitation center was two miles from our home and five miles from Carol's. We wanted our mother nearby so one of us could be there every day to monitor her and help with therapy. Mom couldn't even sit upright without support, and she could not control many of her bodily functions. She also could not swallow safely without aspirating.

Her life had changed so dramatically that it was almost impossible for us to comprehend or bear. But my mother fought desperately to regain her physical strength and control over her body through endless hours of physical, occupational, and speech therapy. Her sheer determination practically wore out the staff. And when the therapists finished their work, I would start mine—having my mother repeat everything she had just done. Some of the exercises to help restore her swallowing reflex were belittling for her, and she would complain when I made her stick out her tongue and wag it from side to side. It would tear at my insides when she begged me for just a drop of water or Italian ice on her tongue. I couldn't imagine what it must have felt like to not be able to drink liquids or eat even a morsel of food. After those sessions, I would go home and clutch Bunny Boy and pray. And sometimes cry. Amazingly, the mouth therapy worked. After six weeks, Mom could eat pureed food and enjoy her favorite drink, a chocolate milkshake.

With all the Buchalski family, our mother had more visitors than any other patient, according to the staff. But we weren't enough.

"When will you bring my grandson over?" she asked one day. She had many grandsons, but I knew *who* she was talking about.

I thought she was kidding. But then I thought, *Why not?*

I brought Bunny Boy over one afternoon. Mom was sitting in her wheelchair outside, under the gazebo with some other patients. By now, she could sit up without any help. As I wheeled Mom around the gardens with Bunny Boy on her lap, the amazing reaction we received from many of the patients was so heartwarming that it occurred to me that I might be onto something. I knew about therapy dogs, but had there ever been a therapy rabbit?

One afternoon, a woman who had not uttered more than one word at a go since her three months at the center strung together four words when I put Bunny Boy on her lap. He licked her hand. "I waaaant thaaaat buuunny," she managed to say, slowly and painfully. It was an amazing moment I will always remember. The staff nearby cheered, amazed by her accomplishment. During another visit, a young gentleman with Down syndrome in a wheelchair touched Bunny Boy's nose and said, "Buuunnny here!" while pointing to his lap. Bunny Boy curled up on his knees, completely trusting the stranger.

Bunny Boy's informal visits quickly became a welcome treat for everyone. Our lagomorph had won the hearts of the patients and the staff. Ultimately, whenever we prepared to leave, someone begged us to come back. And often we did. Not a single member of the staff asked me for any identification or papers showing that Bunny Boy and I were a certified therapy team. They turned a blind eye, grateful for our visits. Somehow, I felt like I had always known that Bunny Boy was meant to bring love and inspiration to many people—not just to me.

By the end of June, my mother had regained control of her bladder and bowels and was able to eat normal food, but even after two months of intense therapy, she failed to meet certain physical therapy requirements. She was deemed "physically non-rehabilitative"—what a horrible word! We were devastated, and we couldn't imagine how Mom felt.

We brought our mother back to the home she loved so much to live out the rest of her days with dignity. Our childhood home became a revolving door as my siblings and her grandchildren visited regularly, a true testament to her well-lived life. My older nieces and nephews would bring along their college-age friends, and Mom would quote Shakespeare, which kept their attention.

In the weeks and months that followed, I spent time with my mother almost every day. On Sundays, Carol and I would wheel her to church for the afternoon mass, weather permitting. About once every two weeks, I would drive Mom up to Mount St. Francis in Ringwood, New Jersey—the summer retreat for the clergy of the Archdiocese of Paterson. Bunny Boy would come along for the ride. For as long as I can remember, my mother found peace and solace strolling the parklike grounds where magnificent four-foot-tall limestone Stations of the Cross stood. The nineteenth-century brick castle sat at the top of a long hill that shadowed Ringwood Manor, the old summer residence of the Cooper family of Cooper Union in Manhattan. Being there brought back wonderful memories from when I was a young girl, when our family used to picnic on the grounds every summer. Bunny Boy would sit on Mom's lap as I pushed her wheelchair along the paths. We'd say the Stations of the Cross as we went along and admire the lush gardens full of day lilies, lavender, azaleas, rhododendrons, and, as summer arrived, annuals like petunias and geraniums. Mom's faith was strong.

Somedays, I would lie next to my mother in her hospital bed and gently massage her pain-ridden back and hip or read to her and tell her how much I loved her. Other times, we would listen to soothing music until she fell asleep. In a strange way, Mom had become like a child. And the more she needed me, the more I wanted to care for her. I simply couldn't imagine life without her. My mother had showed me how to love and care. She taught me how to live a good, faith-filled life. She was everything I strived to be, and over the years, I had tried to follow in her footsteps and give back to the community.

Bunny Boy, too, was showing more apparent signs of aging at a quickening pace. I worried that his second episode of cardiac arrest had sped up the aging process somehow—or maybe I had just been so busy caring for my mother that I had missed the signs. I searched the Internet for "Signs of an Aging Rabbit." Bunny Boy had them all. His appetite was still voracious, but my little buddy looked tired. He had started to sit hunched over while staring into space for short periods of time, instead of sitting upright on his haunches. His skin was starting to sag. He seemed to be losing muscle mass. His activity level had also decreased. The days of bunny NASCAR around the rooms were a distant memory, and the "King of the Castle" chair lay vacant as he spent more of his time hanging out on the floor. He was using his litter pan sporadically. My heart broke when I watched him try to hop in—after failing, he would give up and relieve himself around the perimeter of the pan instead. Bunny Boy had also stopped spraying me. It was heart-wrenching for all of us to watch him—and my mother—slow down.

By late summer, Bunny Boy had become a regular patient at Dr. Welch's office. His facial abscess had moved into his sinus and thick discharge was coming out of his nose—the respiratory infection called "snuffles." Bunny Boy had also developed an abscess on his left hock despite the fact that we had resumed the penicillin injections. It had taken me several months to get over the fear of giving him injections again; we had no choice. Sadly, at this point, we had all made the difficult decision that there would be no more surgeries for Bunny Boy, and because of that we seemed to be losing the battle.

Dr. Welch checked his joints and spine regularly for any obvious signs of arthritis. She found nothing but prescribed an anti-inflammatory just in case to make him more comfortable. The kitchen counters were now crowded with tubes of antibiotic creams. Nasal rinses. Sterile mouth washes. Mounds of bandages and syringes. Prescription bottles. And a large carton of Q-tips. The cotton swabs were indispensable for cleaning out the small holes on Bunny Boy's face and hock. Chris registered his complaint about the Q-tips immediately. "I've been asking for Q-tips for close to a year, and I didn't get a single one. Now Bunny Boy needs Q-tips and he has an economy size box in less than twenty-four hours?"

Dr. Welch would also draw blood at each visit and examine Bunny Boy's jaw, hocks, and his entire body. Fortunately, his jaw still moved fluidly.

"Bunny Boy eats plenty, and he still purrs. He's happy—I know he is," I said during one visit. "I'm not ready to lose him, Dr. Welch."

"Bunny Boy's not going anywhere yet," she replied in her adorable way I'd come to love. "But I'm worried about this abscess on his face."

So was I. The infection seemed to be spreading deeper into his sinus cavity.

"Bunny Boy definitely has some fight left in him," she said. "His weight is stable and his vital signs are strong. Let's switch up the antibiotic and repeat the blood work."

I heaved a sigh of relief. It wasn't time.

"There's always the critical care food if he has a hard time chewing the pellets because his face could be sore," she added. "He can save his energy for more important things like playing or burrowing and doing things that bunnies love to do!" She was right. And who could have ever imagined that I would be hand-feeding my beautiful mother and Bunny Boy at the same time?

It went like this. Bunny Boy and I would sit on the recliner, and he would suck down his breakfast from a syringe while I watched the lively Katie Couric overshadow her male cohost, Matt Lauer, on *The Today Show*. It would take almost forty-five minutes for him to eat the recommended amount. In the evenings, I would feed him another twelve syringes of yummy food while we all watched HBO's *Mad Men*. As Don Draper smoked and drank, Bunny Boy ate his dinner. After two weeks of being hand-fed, if I was not in the playroom by seven in the morning, Bunny Boy would be sitting at the bottom of the stairs waiting patiently for his breakfast. He had decided that his critical care was far more delicious than his old, has-been pellets!

Bunny Boy's patience must have run out one morning. Using his limited strength, he tried to climb up the stairs to my bedroom and sadly slid all the way back down. Chris, visibly upset, came into our room carrying Bunny Boy, describing the thuds he had heard.

Despite his ordeal on the stairs, Bunny Boy lunged from Chris's arms and landed onto my head. He started burrowing in my pillow. "You're still full of life," I whispered into his tall ears as I tucked him under the covers and told him it was too early to play. "We'll eat at a more reasonable hour, Bunny Boy."

The fall brought even sadder days for me. I had already called my siblings and told them that I didn't think Bunny Boy would be with us much longer. Those were very difficult words for me to utter. I had come downstairs one morning to find Bunny Boy lying on his side, kicking his front and back legs wildly, unable to get up. I wondered how long he'd been lying that way. I flew over the baby gate we had set up to keep him safe in the playroom at night and placed him on all fours to see if he could stand up by himself. He teetered for just a second, regained his balance, and hopped onto my lap and started licking my face as if nothing was out of the ordinary.

I called Dr. Welch as soon as their office opened at eight o'clock.

"How will I know when Bunny Boy is close to dying?" I asked, fearful that I might have to put him to sleep at some point.

There was no definitive answer but for his blood work, which would show us if he went into renal failure or congestive heart failure.

"Bunnies have an amazing way of hiding their illnesses. Often until it is too late." I had heard those words before. "Enjoy your time with Bunny Boy," she said warmly. "I'll stay in touch."

Over the years, Dr. Welch had gone above and beyond the call of duty, taking calls from me at the most inopportune times. She always thought nothing of calling me the next day to see how Bunny Boy was doing after we had come in for one thing or another—all while she was raising four children of her own, taking in rescue pets, and mastering any sport or skill that someone said she couldn't do. We loved her.

Bunny Boy's blood work came back fine just one more time. He was not suffering from renal failure or congestive heart failure. He was still playful and didn't seem to be bothered by anything. I knew he was happy.

Eventually, the daily visits to my mother's, Bunny Boy's full regimen of care, and keeping up with the house and food shopping and cooking for a six-foot-one-and-still-growing teen started to take its toll on me. I was finding it difficult to get out of bed in the morning. The stress had wracked my body with intense pain and fatigue. In my place, Ward would head down the stairs every morning to greet Bunny Boy in his usual manner.

"Helloooooo, rabbit. Mommy will be down soon."

One morning, I heard something different. "Hellooo—are you okay, pal?"

I hit the ground running, scaled the gate, and saw Bunny Boy lying on the rug in a way that told me he wasn't right. I lifted him up and placed him on all fours, but he gave up and laid down again. I whisked him up and tucked him tight against my chest. A profound sadness came over us. Bunny Boy had gone from a feisty, utterly adorable kit whose abilities could rival a high jumper, a race car driver, or a break-dancer to a geriatric bunny with horrible bathroom habits and old, rotted teeth in what had seemed like a blink of an eye—but, still, he had endured with an indelible spirit and an amazing will to survive. I was losing him a little more each day, just as I was losing my mother. Mom was now bedridden. Between the two of them, it was a cruel reminder that we all have to grow old.

"You'll let me know somehow when you've had enough, right, pal?" I whispered, wiping away a lone tear.

I swaddled Bunny Boy in his favorite leopard-print blanket and took him up to my bedroom that morning. I canceled my plans for the day. I lay on the bed beside him and just spoke to him. Bunny Boy rested most of the time instead of playing or burrowing. I could see he was tired and weak. I reminded him how he had turned my and my family's world upside down with his loving, quirky, upbeat personality. I told him how proud I was of him for never giving up when life threw him one difficult, humiliating curveball after another. I thanked him for his loyalty and companionship, and for his amazing ability to keep me fighting when things got me down. And I thanked Bunny Boy for helping to save my life.

Chris peeked around the corner when he came home from school.

"Bunny Boy's been going downhill for a while, Mom," he said softly. "But he's had a wonderful life. He's only alive because of the love and care you gave him. We all loved Bunny Boy, but he was your baby."

I glanced at my lanky seventeen-year-old boy and started to sob. He had so eloquently spoken the words my broken heart needed to hear.

A few days later, Julie came home from college for a long weekend. She laid out the Phi Sigma Sigma sorority crafts she was making for her "little" on her bed next to Bunny Boy, gluing and coloring while she sang him his favorite reggae tune over and over again, tenderly. He slept instead of pillaging her supplies. But they were together. Julie seemed to be preparing herself for the inevitable.

One night, the four of us sat around the family room's coffee table, looking through photo albums and jokingly counting Bunny Boy's pictures while he was curled up in a ball on Ward's chest. Suddenly, Bunny Boy looked so small. We read the *Suburban News* article together, Bunny Boy's claim to fame. And we played poker with the deck of Bunny Boy cards.

Halloween passed and the first frost set in. Bunny Boy's appetite remained robust. His loss of physical strength failed to dull his spirit. He seemed quite content resting in his cozy warren in the lagomorph lounge. But I was becoming distressed as I watched him slow down. I knew my time with him was running out. I didn't have the faintest idea how to prepare myself—so I didn't. Instead, I just spent more time with him, lying beside him on the sofa or on the floor—wherever Bunny Boy felt more comfortable. I would kiss his tall ears and twittering nose and tell him how much I loved him. Some nights, we would lie together until one or two in the morning before I would go upstairs to get some sleep. Some nights I would go to bed around eleven o'clock and come back down to the lagomorph lounge around three o'clock to check on him and cuddle some more.

There was one night in particular I will cherish forever. I laid Bunny Boy on his side, across my chest, while Ward and I sat in bed watching the eleven o'clock news. His head was facing Ward. After about ten minutes, he used what little strength he had left to lift his body and reposition himself so he was lying on his stomach with his head looking directly up at me. I leaned down and met his eyes. We stayed that way until my neck was too sore. Quietly, Ward got up and slept in Julie's room.

I would soon realize the significance of that special moment. Though I didn't know how to say my goodbyes, Bunny Boy was preparing to say his.

• • •

It was Sunday, November 15. I had just returned home from mass. Bunny Boy seemed to be zoned out. The first thought that struck me was that this was the end. I knew that Kelly and Tanya worked on Sundays at the Franklin Lakes Animal Hospital, caring for the boarded animals even though the hospital was closed. Ward and I drove Bunny Boy over, entering by the back entrance. Kelly checked him over carefully and administered some intravenous fluids. Iron Bunny perked up, as if he had just been given a mocha latte instead of saline. I was confused. His breathing was normal and Kelly could not hear any heart irregularities. He was not in congestive heart failure.

"Sometimes when animals begin to go into renal failure, they don't drink. Bunny Boy was dehydrated. You can leave him here until Dr. Welch comes in tomorrow morning or you can bring him home and call when we open tomorrow. One of us will be here all night."

I couldn't leave Bunny Boy there. I had to be with him.

"Bunny Boy's fought a long, tough battle," Kelly said with a smile before we left.

At home that night, I fed Bunny Boy his critical care food, some pureed apples, and melted yogurt drops. I indulged him with all of his favorite things. When he was finished, he hopped on top of one of his old wicker bunny tunnels behind the sofa and looked straight at us for a moment. As if he was trying to tell us that he was still okay. I wiggled my nose up against his.

"I didn't know you still had it in you, little man."

It would be Bunny Boy's last hurrah.

Ward was the first to go downstairs that dreadful next morning.

"Come down right away, Nance."

The night before, I had gone to bed around three a.m. Chris later told us that he had peeked in on Bunny Boy around five a.m. when he got up to go to the bathroom. Bunny Boy had been curled up like a fetus on the rug. I wish he had woken me up.

I jumped out of bed. Ward was holding Bunny Boy. He gave him to me immediately. There was no moisture or pink color left in Bunny Boy's nose. His eyes were sunken. His body was limp, and it lacked its usual warmth. His fur looked strangely dull, almost straggly.

"He's dying," I wailed, tucking him under my robe. It was seven thirty.

"It's okay, Bunny Boy, Mommy knows you have had enough," I whimpered. "I understand if you're ready."

My precious boy and I locked eyes. He let out two small scratchy squeals, several seconds apart. Then, his head fell back slightly, his thumper legs extended outward, and Bunny Boy took his last breath—cradled in my arms.

My five-pound bundle of joy had finally given up.

We drove to Dr. Welch's office with Bunny Boy wrapped in his old leopard blanket. I was still in my bathrobe. I was unable to cry—not yet. I hung onto Bunny Boy for dear life. Dr. Welch was absent that day, gone away for a few days with her family. Kat, another technician, put a stethoscope to his chest and made it official. Bunny Boy had passed to the other side of the Rainbow Bridge.

That's when my faucets opened—and they didn't stop. My tears flowed onto Bunny Boy's lifeless body as I told him how much I loved him and how much I would miss him.

"I can't believe today has really come, Mrs. Laracy," Kelly remarked softly. "We all got used to Bunny Boy making it through everything. He was a good sport and a real fighter."

"He was," Ward managed to say.

"You were such a good boy, silly," I blubbered. "You were my inspiration, you beautiful, crazy, little animal. What am I going to do without you?"

I spent those final moments loving my bunny, thanking God for the miracle of his entire life.

"He waited for you, Nance," Ward said, wrapping his arms around me and kissing my teary cheek. "You got your wish." And I had. Bunny Boy had died in the warm, safe embrace of my arms.

We gave Kat instructions to have Bunny Boy cremated individually instead of together with a group of other animals, as vets sometimes do. Then I handed my little boy over to Kelly, as I had done so many times before. Only this time, Bunny Boy wouldn't be coming back.

•   •   •

I walked into the house in a daze. I looked up the foyer stairs toward the lagomorph lounge and ran up and sat in the recliner where I had fed Bunny Boy for the past four months and spent countless nights with him on my lap. It didn't seem possible that Bunny Boy was gone. I grabbed our special pillow and hugged it. It was still covered with some dried food and strands of his fur.

Chris poked his head out of his room. "I'm so sorry, Mom. I miss Bunny Boy already." Then he closed the door to grieve in his own teenage way.

I called Julie. Bunny Boy's number-two girl was at a loss for words. Then I called Donna, who was at my front door in ten minutes. We sat on the sofa and reminisced about some of our fondest memories with Bunny Boy, in particular, the day we had been mistaken as a couple at the AMC.

I looked around the room at all of Bunny Boy's things—his toys, his bowls, his wicker tunnel. The lagomorph lounge would never be the same.

"It is going to take a long time, Nance," said Donna, reaching for my hand.

"It was like losing a baby, Donna."

"You nursed him for almost nine years," she said kindly. "He *was* your baby."

"That's what made Bunny Boy so special. He needed me as much as I needed him."

Early that afternoon, I drove to my mother's. We laid together in her hospital bed and she wrapped her frail, thin arms around me.

"I really loved that rabbit," she whispered, kissing my cheek.

It seemed like just yesterday that my mother had shown up at five thirty in the morning to drive into New York with Bunny Boy and me, when I was so sick.

"I need to know that Bunny Boy is okay, Mom—that he's peaceful."

"Bunny Boy's with your father now, sweetheart," she said. I prayed he was.

When Carol came home from work, we cried together and talked about her rabbit babysitting days. Boarding Bunny Boy at their house shortly after their own cat and dog had died was just the therapy they needed at the time.

Finally, I visited Loretta at Scuffy's.

"I should have stayed with Bunny Boy the whole night," I said tearfully, regretfully. "I didn't know he was dying."

I could see her trying to hide her own tears. "Bunny Boy didn't want you to see him at the end," she reassured. "He wanted you to remember him the way he was."

"But he was alone. I would have—"

"Bunny Boy died in your arms. That's what's important."

There was something important I needed to express. "I need to know that Bunny Boy is happy. That he's okay," I said, once again.

"Bunny Boy had a wonderful life. He lived longer than most healthy rabbits."

I reached into my pocket and handed Loretta one of my favorite pictures of Bunny Boy, which I usually kept it in the glove compartment of my car. Bunny Boy was sitting on the "King of the Castle" chair with his wicker ball. He couldn't have been more than three years old. I said a teary goodbye to Loretta and the rest of the staff and started down the windy road toward home.

I drove through the darkness, my eyesight blurred by my tears.

Visions of Bunny Boy as a kit flashed through my mind. The days of litter training and chewing. The days of youthful binkying and pranks. When I turned the corner onto our street, it seemed darker than usual. I flipped on my high beams—and, out of nowhere, a bunny dashed across the bright stream of light from the lawn on one side of the road, stopping in the middle of the asphalt. He looked at me through my windshield, much like a deer caught in headlights. For a second, I thought I had imagined it. I quickly put the car in park and stared at the bunny. He hopped closer to the car bumper and looked at me more intently, as if he felt my gaze. Then, without further ado, he scampered off into the woods, free as a bird.

I pulled over to the side of the road and called Ward, shivering.

"It was a sign from Bunny Boy, Ward," I exclaimed. "I must have said at least four times today that I needed to know that Bunny Boy was okay." Ward uttered a few comforting words. I could hear the sadness in his voice. I looked far into the woods for the bunny. Somehow, amid my sadness, a sense of relief filled me. Bunny Boy had let me know that he was fine.

That bunny sighting was the first of several amazing coincidences and miracles yet to come after Bunny Boy's passing.

• • •

That night, I walked upstairs to my bedroom around eleven. My bed looked like a drop-off center for unwanted stuffed bunnies. Ward had piled up every stuffed bunny we had from all over the house on my side of the bed in an attempt to cheer me up. I fell into the pool of fake fur—and cried. Not for long, but intensely. I curled up in the fetal position, clutching my all-time favorite stuffed rabbit—a sandy-colored bunny with white ears that doubled as a puppet. Julie and Chris had surprised me with it one year for Mother's Day.

I lay awake, torturing myself for going to sleep the day before during Bunny Boy's last night. My stomach was turning in knots. Excuses and should-haves kept me awake. Sleep never came. Around three in the morning, I went down to the lagomorph lounge and sat in the recliner. This time, I wrapped myself in Bunny Boy's leopard blanket. I longed for my father's voice, his warm smile.

"Take good care of my boy, Dad," I said.

I returned to bed a second time, clutching Bunny Boy's blanket. The next thing I knew, I felt a soft tap on my head. It was seven thirty in the morning. I had slept past my usual alarm, which Ward had turned off when he saw I was finally sleeping.

Chris was standing at the edge of my bed, holding a checkered gift bag.

"This was left on the front porch," he whispered. I unwrapped the lavender floral tissue paper, and inside was a life-size stuffed rabbit that looked just like Bunny Boy. It was eerie. The bunny was sitting on its haunches with its ears straight up—happy ears. My friend Mary Beth had dropped the package off on her way to work. The faucets opened again. I was unable to stop—I didn't want to.

My new stuffed bunny was the beginning of an extremely touching tribute to Bunny Boy that I will never forget, from all who knew him. Those first few days, baskets of flowers and plants arrived at my door. Some of them were in ceramic bunny planters, others had bunnies of one type or another perched among the greenery. The UPS man came twice one day, bringing large and small stuffed bunnies in pastel colors and the more traditional shades of brown, white, or gray. Perhaps the most meaningful gesture was when the neighbor's fifteen-year-old daughter dropped off her favorite childhood bunny to comfort me—on loan.

My foyer became a shrine for Bunny Boy. The surgical staff at Estes Park Hospital in Colorado, where Tom worked as a nurse, sent beautiful cards with inspirational words, saying they felt as if they had all known Bunny Boy. The story of my brother's heroic effort to revive Bunny Boy had circulated throughout his hospital, and the *Suburban News* feature article hung proudly in his office.

I wasn't alone for more than a few hours those first few days. Friends, neighbors, and family members came by with cups of coffee, my favorite chocolate iced donuts, and dinners for a grieving mommy. I might as well have been sitting Shiva, just without the bagels and fish platters. Donna, in her delicate way, had many spiritual words to share with me. Employees from the Franklin Lakes Animal Hospital also called. Dr. Welch was heartbroken when she returned from her vacation.

"I lived and breathed for Bunny Boy," she said, her voice cracking. "We gave him the long life he deserved. Bunny Boy fought when he shouldn't have had the strength. Mrs. Laracy—you know that, right?"

While Dr. Welch cared for every pet with the same love and tender care, Bunny Boy was her pride and joy. And she wasn't shy about admitting to that. She and the Animal Medical Center had kept Bunny Boy alive about eight years more than anyone could have expected, while at the same time making sure he had the best quality of life.

The staff at the Animal Medical Center was also deeply saddened by the news of Bunny Boy's passing. Dr. Quesenberry thanked me personally for the role Bunny Boy played in rabbit medicine. During the near decade we had Bunny Boy, the hospital had made great strides when it came to medical care for bunnies. Rabbits had become the pet du jour in large cities; in particular, Manhattan. Suddenly, bunny patients were plentiful. More accurate statistics regarding the prognosis for medical procedures performed on bunnies were now available. Rabbits were on the radar!

There was nothing more I could have asked for. I felt incredibly blessed.

Now I would simply need time to adjust to the loss of my best friend.

Chapter 31

Reality set in. I found myself wandering around the house like a lost soul, talking to Bunny Boy as if he were still there. I ached inside and out. I felt numb and lethargic. Everywhere I looked, there were reminders of Bunny Boy. The baskets of medical supplies were still on the kitchen counter, alongside half empty bottles of antibiotics and pain medicine that were labelled: "Bunny Boy Laracy 668 Dakota/BUNNY Trail, Franklin Lakes." ("Bunny Trail" was Dr. Welch's idea.) The lagomorph lounge was still exactly the same way as it was the day Bunny Boy died. The wicker tunnel he sat on the night before was still by the couch, and his pillow and blanket were on the recliner.

It had been four long days, and I knew it was time to distract myself. I tried to get onto the computer to continue writing my book, but it was too painful. So, Ward and I made a last-minute decision to go ahead with our on-again, off-again weekend to the Finger Lakes of New York with our friends Keith and Michele, which we had planned back in September.

Keith and Michele arrived early Saturday morning, their usual cheerful selves. They handed me a small package wrapped in gold glitter paper. Inside was a beautiful hand-painted ceramic Christmas bunny ornament. We shared hugs, coffee, and bagels before hitting the road. The Finger Lakes were about five hours away.

I tried to keep the conversation in the car light, at least initially, until Michele mentioned that I needed to grieve properly. That was a license to cry. In between my tears, one Bunny Boy story or special moment after another kept us occupied for much of the trip.

I tried to sum it up. "Bunny Boy was no ordinary rabbit. He was the breath of fresh air that blew into my life when I needed it the most. He was a beloved member of our family for the near decade we were lucky enough to have him. Bunny Boy filled a void no one else could fill. Like a cat, he seemed to have nine lives, surviving one medical calamity after another. He was downright mischievous and utterly charming. His loyalty and complete trust in me were unwavering. Bunny Boy loved deeply without discriminating, and he touched the souls of all he met with his gentle spirit and endearing nature. He was made of iron. When his body was failing, he fought to hold onto life—savoring every minute. Bunny Boy loved a simple ride in the car, a silly game, or an afternoon on the porch. He wanted to be loved. And he returned that love unconditionally. Bunny Boy left his mark on the medical community worldwide, but most of all he helped save my life in more ways than one. He was, in the end, my role model for how to conduct oneself with dignity when life throws you one curveball after another."

We arrived at our lodging in Lake Skaneateles, the easternmost part of the Finger Lakes. The quaint inn, which had served as an old stagecoach stop in the 1800s, was located on the main street across from the lake. The exterior was colonial blue with black shutters. The lobby boasted a large stone fireplace, tapestry Queen Anne chairs, and a deep-green wood-framed velvet sofa. I pictured Bunny Boy nestled on one of the chairs and felt my eyes gloss over. Sconces lit the rustic foyer and a crooked pine staircase led up to the guest rooms.

I was unable to sleep much that first night at the inn. I missed Bunny Boy terribly. I longed for him; I thought about life without him. I would miss our special time on the front porch; I would miss having him as my traveling companion. I would miss being scampered on and gently licked during a good snuggle. There would be no more rubbing noses or silly antics or mischief. The house would be too calm and quiet without him underfoot.

The following morning, we met our friends in the main dining room for a buffet breakfast. In an attempt to drown my sorrows, I carb-loaded, devouring two chocolate chip muffins, a croissant with butter, and a toasted bagel with jelly.

The weather was winterlike, the water dull beneath the gray skies. We toured the remaining points of interest of Lake Skaneateles and made our way to Lake Seneca by late morning. The upstate towns were lacking tourists and the absence of sun cast a looming shadow over the entire region. We stopped at different wineries to sample their selections of red and white wines. A tide of emotion came over me at winery number six when a very old chocolate Labrador with three legs came limping out from behind the tasting bar. His entire snout was framed with gray hair. He had lost his back leg from cancer when he was only three years old. As I petted him, I could see Bunny Boy, unable to get up off the hardwood floors, and I simply had to tell my story to the proprietor while I tasted yet another three wines, which only made me more emotional.

At the next winery, I was hit with a rush of wooziness. It was almost two o'clock and the only thing we had eaten since breakfast were a few crackers, some cheese, and nuts. We decided to lunch at the Harbor Inn in Watkins Glen. The waitress walked us to a table in the bar area overlooking the lake. I glanced over the menu quickly, picked my salad, and began to torture myself again—wondering why I hadn't stayed up with Bunny Boy that very last night.

"I need to take a walk by myself for a few minutes," I told Ward and our friends.

I strolled aimlessly down the brightly lit marble corridors of the hotel, talking to Bunny Boy. I still couldn't believe he had left me. I gazed out of the windows toward the lake and the dreariness of the bare trees, the black water, and the ragged underbrush, which seemed to swallow me up. I must have looked lost, because I soon heard, "Are you looking for the ladies' room?"

I shook my head politely and continued walking to a "T" in the hallway, when I stopped abruptly. On the wall in front of me were four blown-up landscapes of Lake Seneca from the 1920s. The fifth photo, which was flanked by the other four, showed a small cement structure with a large sign that read "BUNNY'S PLACE." I stood for a moment, reading the description beneath the large letters.

Bunny's Place was a snack bar located across the street from Lakeside

Park on Route 414. With the witty motto of "If you are hungry, don't go by," how could anyone not want to support the business?

It seemed like an uncanny coincidence. A sudden lightheartedness came over me. I felt Bunny Boy's presence. I ran back to the bar to get my traveling therapy group to show off my discovery.

"We were sent here for a reason," I whispered to Michele as I took several pictures of the unique historic photograph.

I was in a much better mood for the rest of the day. The four of us laughed and joked over the silliest things like a bunch of college kids. During dinner, a blues singer kept my mind from wandering to Bunny Boy for at least an hour—a new record—while I enjoyed a French onion soup paired with grilled scallops on a bed of greens, the perfect culinary delight for the cold, weary traveler—me. When we retired to the grand room, we found a group of older gentlemen from Albany engaged in a boisterous discussion about the existence of God. It was certainly the wrong time for anybody to bring up the possibility of no god in my presence, and out of respect for my faith and Bunny Boy's death, Ward and Keith, the two agnostics out of the four of us, chose to keep silent.

We retired for the night. The pilot light from the gas fireplace was the only light source when we walked through the door of our room; housekeeping had pulled the heavy drapes closed. Sadness enveloped me again. I pushed back the feeling and flipped on all of the lights and the radio. I sat in bed reading a select few chapters from my manuscript—the sillier ones—until I could barely keep my eyes open. I pulled the covers up and around me and fell asleep.

The next morning, we enjoyed a delicious breakfast and sipped coffee by the windows on the sun porch while discussing the day's plans. A smile softened my face when I noticed a mother duck and her six babies floating along Lake Skaneateles. I imagined Bunny Boy as a kit. It felt so good to smile.

With the blazing sun overhead, the panoramic view of Lake Cayuga, our next stop, was warm and inviting. The blue skies changed hue as different clusters of clouds passed over. Around mid-afternoon, we came across the MacKenzie-Childs farmhouse and factory store on the north shore of Lake Cayuga—a destination that Keith and Ward had penciled a large red X over on our map, identifying it under "Things not to visit." MacKenzie-Childs is a high-end retail manufacturer of unique, colorful, and often whimsical furniture and home accessories.

"We can skip the store," I said, "But please, we *must* take the house tour." How could Ward possibly turn me down after all that had happened the previous week? Interior decorating was one of my passions. I had literally chosen every fabric sample, rug, paint color, and accessory for our own home and even helped several of my friends with theirs. Under duress, the men agreed to go on a tour of the farmhouse.

We purchased our tickets and waited in the foyer with a dozen or so other tourists. A petite blonde girl who looked to be in her early twenties walked in wearing a pair of Victorian-style MacKenzie-Childs slippers that I recognized from their catalog. She had on a pink cashmere sweater and a navy-blue pencil skirt.

"Good afternoon, ladies and gentlemen," she said, starting the tour. "Please notice when you tour our farmhouse today that MacKenzie-Childs uses similar color schemes and many unique patterns throughout the house according to certain motifs. And one of our favorite motifs is bunnies!"

Michele nudged me before I could react.

"This bunny stuff is a little strange, Nance, don't you think?"

"Just a little," I replied.

Our group moved slowly from the foyer into the dining room. The cottage-style windows had patterned draperies with soft pink, bright raspberry, and white as their predominant colors—as did the dining room chairs. I almost gasped when I saw the magnificent glass top coffee table in the corner of the room. The base was made of four shimmering life-sized porcelain bunnies, hooked together as if they were dancing. My heart melted when I got up close, taking in each detail of the enchanting work of art.

When we shuffled into the living room my eye was immediately drawn to two matching needlepoint pillows on the sofa, featuring bunnies nibbling on flowers in a garden. They gave me chills. I reached for Ward's hand.

"Can you believe this, honey?"

And the bunny aura continued.

The girl's bedroom on the second floor had a bright yellow, pink, and green checked bedspread with yellow trellising vines along the border, almost like a picture frame. On the shabby chic bedside tables sat two white porcelain bunny lamps the size of our Bunny Boy. The bunnies had delicately painted blue eyes and pink noses. The lampshades were exquisitely trimmed with pastel pink beading. *I must have one of those lamps*, I thought to myself.

It was strangely therapeutic walking through a farmhouse full of bunny-themed items. "I forgot my wallet back at the Inn, Nance," Ward joked, as if I might not have mine.

Despite our initial agreement, Michele and I barged through the door of the warehouse store and began exploring the fifteen thousand feet of drywall that stocked MacKenzie-Childs furniture, lamps, dinnerware, glassware, linens, drapes, notions, footwear, and candles. It was like heaven on earth. Ward and Keith parked themselves on a bench to answer emails. Soon, I noticed the very same bunny lamp out of the corner of my eye.

"There it is, Michele," I said. "The Lamp." It was even dreamier up close.

Suddenly, I heard a soft, sweet voice coming from behind me. "Do you like that lamp?" I looked over my shoulder. A darling girl, about ten years old, was standing next to a woman I assumed was her mother. She had cropped sandy brown hair and deep brown eyes.

"I love it!" I said, curious as to why she had asked.

"We're getting a bunny tomorrow," the girl blurted out. "I've always wanted a bunny."

I nearly dropped the pair of Victorian slippers I had been holding onto. I couldn't help but wonder why I was here, at this very spot, in this very moment.

"Are you really getting a bunny tomorrow?" I asked, looking at the woman.

"We are."

"Are you her mom?"

"Sort of," the woman replied sadly. "I'm her aunt." I could tell by the young girl's expression that there was a part of the story I might not ever know. "She's always wanted a pet of her own," the woman added, looking at her niece fondly. "My husband is allergic to dogs and cats, so we thought we would buy a bunny."

"I'd like to tell you about my own bunny," I suddenly stuttered. "But before I do, please promise me you won't keep your bunny outside the house in one of those hutches!"

"My husband just painted the hutch yesterday," said the woman, surprised. "Why wouldn't we keep the bunny in the hutch?"

"You can and should train your bunny to live in the house like a dog or cat," I said, probably with too much of an authoritative tone. The idea of any rabbit living in a hutch sickened me now. I softened my voice. "Come, let's sit here." We sat down on a colorful striped ottoman in the hallway. For the next few minutes, I gave them pointers on how to house-train and raise their bunny-to-be, most likely providing more instructions than they wanted to hear. Then, I told them the abridged version of Bunny Boy's nine-year stay on this earth—up until the moment he died in my arms. It was like a pipe had burst and all the water had come gushing out. I couldn't help myself. A feeling of happiness rather than sadness came over me as I spoke about my beloved bunny.

The young girl was jubilant. She was bouncing on the ottoman and twirling the strands of her hair with her fingers. At that moment, I knew this bunny was meant to be.

We said our goodbyes, and Michele and I hugged each other, acknowledging the amazing coincidence of the little girl and her aunt. How could we not? We practically ran to find Ward and Keith, who were standing at the far end of the store, waiting to show us the same bunny table we had seen on the tour. Ward had stumbled upon it while searching for the men's room.

"It's simply unbelievable!" Michele said to Ward and Keith.

"We thought so, too!" they replied, referring to the table, which was truly exquisite.

"No, not that! I mean this young girl who came out of nowhere and told us she happens to be buying a bunny tomorrow."

With great detail and emotion, I shared our story. Both Ward and Keith were visibly moved.

"I believe the girl's mother might have died," I said. "She needs this bunny."

"Would you like the bunny table or the lamp for Christmas?" Ward asked.

Normally I would have jumped at the offer. But instead, I said, "Thank you, but I'm not sure."

Something far more important was on my mind. I couldn't help but wonder why I had met this young girl. I was deep in thought when I felt a soft tap on my shoulder—it was her!

"Excuse me. I'm sorry to bother you, but can you please tell me the name of your bunny? I would like to name my rabbit after him," she announced proudly.

I threw my arms around her and looked up toward heaven.

"His name was Bunny Boy—and Fluffett, when we thought he was a girl."

"My name is Amy."

I held her small body tight against me.

"You have given me the gift of a lifetime, Amy," I said. "Bunny Boy's spirit will live on in your bunny."

Amy blushed and smiled at us. I cupped her delicate face with my hands. "You're a very special little girl whom I was meant to meet. You see, I'm writing a book about Bunny Boy's life, and I wasn't sure how to end it."

"This is a magnificent ending to a beautiful story," Michelle added. "Bunny Boy is still working his magic."

Indeed, he had. Bunny Boy had gone full circle.

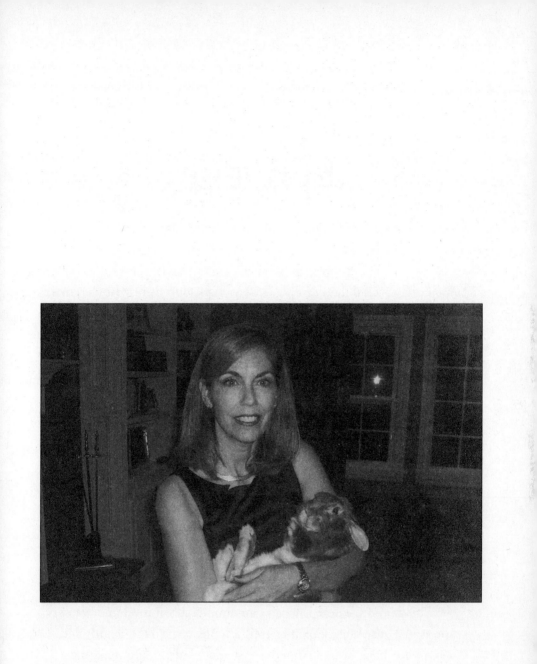

Epilogue

The Friday after Thanksgiving, I went to pick up Bunny Boy's remains from the Franklin Lakes Animal Hospital. As I walked through the door without the usual beautiful bundle in my arms, I took in the familiar surroundings—the bookshelves filled with novels about pets, the cages of rescue kittens, and the tropical fish tank. Bunny Boy and I had spent so much time there. That chapter of my life was now over.

Donna handed me a small mahogany box and a white envelope. Inside the envelope was a card with Bunny Boy's name inscribed beneath the meaningful words, "A Final Act of Love." Underneath that was a beautiful meditation, entitled "The Rainbow Bridge":

Because of its many colors, the bridge connecting Heaven and Earth has come to be known as the Rainbow Bridge. Just this side of the Bridge, there is a land of meadows, hills and lush green valleys. When a beloved pet dies, this wonderful place serves as their new home. There is always an abundance of food and water and warm sunshine. Old and frail animals are young again, and those who have been maimed are made whole. They make new friends and play all day.

There is one thing missing from these carefree surroundings though. The companionship of their loving masters. Time passes and soon another day comes when one of them is distracted by a familiar scent. With nose twitching, ears at attention and eyes staring in delight, this one runs from the group . . . YOU have been seen!

As you embrace, your face is kissed again and again and again, and once more you look into the eyes of your loyal companion. You cross the Rainbow Bridge together, never again to be separated.

We can only hope . . .

Before I left the hospital, my ears perked up to a familiar tune that was playing on the radio.

"Listen to the radio!" I told everyone. "That's my father's song, 'Moon River'!"

On the drive here, I had spoken to him—as I always did—asking for his advice and help. I now knew for certain that Bunny Boy was fine on the other side of the Rainbow Bridge.

My beautiful mother passed away from pneumonia the spring after Bunny Boy died. During that incredibly difficult time, I did a lot of soul searching amidst my grieving. I had thought that I could never have another rabbit or animal companion as special as Bunny Boy, but eight months after my mother's death, a female Jersey Wooly rabbit named Muffin entered my life.

Muffin helped to heal my heart, filling Bunny Boy's huge paw prints. She would come to leave her own distinct mark on the world in a very different way. Inspired by the way Bunny Boy had comforted the residents of Oakland Rehabilitation Center, I started my own 501(c)(3) charity as the first bunny therapy team in the northeast region for Bunnies in Baskets, a pet therapy organization based in Oregon—and Muffin became the essence of my being and my work.

Once we were certified as a therapy team, we visited several nursing homes in the area. When the tragic events in Sandy Hook Elementary in Newtown, Connecticut, occurred, I was contacted by the director of the daycare center and nursery school that shared their driveway. I quickly drove up to Newtown with Muffin in tow and a car full of gifts and presents from our community—a few bunny books from our local library, a bunny craft for the children to do, and chocolate bunny lollipops from a local candy shop. It was a day that will be forever etched in my mind. Our healing power was tremendous.

Within months of our first therapy assignment with the children of Sandy Hook, several other organizations dealing with sick and disabled children contacted me. Our town librarian referred me to Camp Dream Street, an organization in New Jersey that organizes a summer camp for children with cancer. Then CancerCare, a national organization, saw Muffin and me visiting patients at the Christian Healthcare Center in Wyckoff, New Jersey, and asked to meet with me. The Butterflies Program, a children's hospice program out of Valley Hospital in Ridgewood, New Jersey, also approached me at the facility that same day. I began planning bunny-esque therapy programs for both of their organizations. Word spread quickly and I soon found myself designing and implementing programs for the Spring Lake Toy Foundation and the Friendship Circle, other organizations in the New Jersey area that served sick and disabled children.

I continued doing those programs until the fall of 2017 when Muffin died of congestive heart failure due to old age. She was seven years old, her life expectancy. I remain involved with all the charities, simply in another capacity.

Tragically, Dr. Cheryl Welch passed away from metastatic pancreatic cancer about a year after we bought Muffin. She was forty-five. She was diagnosed seemingly out of the blue and lived only seven weeks from the date of her diagnosis. Cheryl left behind four children and a bustling veterinary practice, a huge loss to all. The tribute to her legacy throughout the community and county was astounding and well-deserved. She was truly special in everything she did during her life and posthumously, leaving her mark on the veterinary community with her innovative mind and wonderful people skills.

• • •

After Julie graduated from college, she became a teacher for underserved children in Philadelphia where she met her husband. She is now married with an infant daughter. Chris graduated from college with a degree in chemistry, and Ward is thriving, as busy as ever, in his same job as a lawyer.

As for me, I am now a proud grandmother, and I continue my advocacy work for the chronic pain and animal assisted therapy communities —though without either of my amazing bunnies. I am now dealing with a third painful disease, an autoimmune disease called ankylosing spondylitis. Like Bunny Boy, I am coping with this additional curveball thrown in my path, hopefully with as much dignity, determination, and grace as he did.

Acknowledgments

I want to thank Dr. Cheryl Welch and all the dedicated employees of the Franklin Lakes Animal Hospital who loved and cared for Bunny Boy over the nine years that he lived. I would also like to thank Dr. Welch for encouraging me to write this book—she had faith that I would follow the project through to the end. I would also like to thank Dr. Quesenberry, Dr. Hess, and all of the employees at the Animal Medical Center in New York for their wonderful care and faith in Bunny Boy's resolve. Thank you for allowing Bunny Boy to be part of cutting-edge medical treatment for rabbits.

To my editor, Kim Lim, who fell in love with the story from the first day she read it, thank you for making my words flow beautifully without changing the essence of the book! And thank you for being such a pleasure to work with. To Skyhorse Publishing—thank you for having the faith and foresight to publish a book from a first-time author with a remarkable story to tell.

Finally, I want to thank my family for their love and support during this project, which began over ten years ago, and in particular my beloved mother who insisted that I could do anything, including writing a book. I am sorry, Mom, that you are not here to see the book completed.